Pain Management
PreTest® Self-Assessment and Review

• NOTICE •

Medicine is an ever-changing science. As new research and clinical experience broaden our knowledge, changes in treatment and drug therapy are required. The authors and the publisher of this work have checked with sources believed to be reliable in their efforts to provide information that is complete and generally in accord with the standards accepted at the time of publication. However, in view of the possibility of human error or changes in medical sciences, neither the authors, nor the publisher, nor any other party who has been involved in the preparation or publication of this work warrants that the information contained herein is in every respect accurate or complete, and they are not responsible for any errors or omissions or for the results obtained from use of such information. Readers are encouraged to confirm the information contained herein with other sources. For example and in particular, readers are advised to check the product information sheet included in the package of each drug they plan to administer to be certain that the information contained in this book is accurate and that changes have not been made in the recommended dose or in the contraindications for administration. This recommendation is of particular importance in connection with new or infrequently used drugs.

Pain Management

PreTest® Self-Assessment and Review

Cynthia H. Kahn, M.D.
Department of Anesthesia
Harvard Medical School
Cambridge, Massachusetts

John M. DeSio, M.D.
Princeton Pain Management Center
Princeton, New Jersey

McGraw-Hill, Inc.
Health Professions Division
PreTest® Series

New York   St. Louis   San Francisco   Auckland   Bogotá
Caracas   Lisbon   London   Madrid   Mexico City   Milan   Montreal
New Delhi   San Juan   Singapore   Sydney   Tokyo   Toronto

McGraw-Hill
A Division of The McGraw·Hill Companies

Pain Management: PreTest® Self-Assessment and Review
Copyright © 1996 by McGraw-Hill, Inc. All rights reserved. Printed in the United States of America. Except as permitted under the United States Copyright Act of 1976, no part of this publication may be reproduced or distributed in any form or by any means, or stored in a data base or retrieval system without the prior written permission of the publisher.

1 2 3 4 5 6 7 8 9 0 MALMAL 9 9 8 7 6

ISBN 0-07-052079-8

The editors were Gail Gavert and Bruce MacGregor.
The production supervisors were Clara B. Stanley and Anna Lieggi.
Malloy Lithographers was printer and binder.
This book was set in Times Roman by V&M Graphics.

This book is printed on acid-free paper.

All figures are from the Princeton Pain Management
  Center, Princeton, New Jersey.

Library of Congress Cataloging-in-Publication Data

Kahn, Cynthia H.
    Pain Management : PreTest self-assessment and review /
  Cynthia H. Kahn, John M. DeSio.
        p.   cm.
    Includes bibliographical references.
    ISBN 0-07-052079-8 (alk. paper)
    1. Pain—Treatment—Examinations, questions, etc, 2. Analgesia—
Examinations, questions, etc,   I. DeSio, John M.   II. Title.
      [DNLM: 1. Pain—therapy—examination questions. 2. Palliative
Treatment—examination questions.   WL 18.2 K12c 1996]
RB127.K25   1996
616.1'2305—dc20
DNLM/DLC
for Library of Congress   95-25774

Contents

Preface vii

Introduction ix

Abbreviations xi

Anatomy and Physiology
 Questions 1
 Answers, Explanations, and References 14

Diagnostic Testing
 Questions 29
 Answers, Explanations, and References 33

Types of Pain
 Questions 37
 Answers, Explanations, and References 53

Pain Assessment
 Questions 71
 Answers, Explanations, and References 73

Pharmacology
 Questions 75
 Answers, Explanations, and References 87

Medical and Surgical Techniques of Pain Management
 Questions 101
 Answers, Explanations, and References 119

Pain Management in Pediatric, Critical Care, and Obstetric Populations
 Questions 135
 Answers, Explanations, and References 139

Psychological Aspects of Pain
 Questions 145
 Answers, Explanations, and References 149

Compensation, Disability Assessment, and Medicolegal Issues
 Questions 153
 Answers, Explanations, and References 157

Bibliography 161

Preface

This book has been designed to introduce you to the areas of knowledge covered in the pain certification examinations. At present, three organizations offer certification examinations:

The American Board of Anesthesiology (ABA) provides a Certificate of Added Qualifications in Pain Management to board-certified anesthesiologists with a current medical license who have had 12 months of formal training in acute, chronic, and cancer pain management. Individual exceptions may be made for those who have practiced pain medicine full-time for at least 2 years or half-time for at least 4 years prior to September 1, 1993. The ABA examination is given every other year, usually in the fall. It consists of 200 questions that must be answered during a 4-h period. Multiple true-false (K-type) and one best answer (A-type) questions as well as radiographs and other figures may be present on the examination. There is no oral segment. The Certificate of Added Qualifications in Pain Management is valid for 10 years, after which recertification is required. The current content distribution is 10 to 15 percent anatomy, 10 to 15 percent physiology, 5 to 10 percent pathophysiology, 20 to 25 percent pharmacology, 15 to 20 percent diagnosis of pain states, 20 to 25 percent pain therapy, 2 to 5 percent pediatrics, 1 to 2 percent critical care medicine, 1 to 2 percent costs of medical care, and 1 to 2 percent record keeping. For a full content outline and more information regarding this examination, contact the American Board of Anesthesiology, 100 Constitution Plaza, Hartford, CT 06103. The phone number is (203) 522-9857 and the fax number is (203) 522-6626.

The American Board of Pain Medicine (ABPM) provides a yearly, 8-h, 400-question written examination to doctors of medicine and doctors of osteopathy with a valid medical license and certification by the American Board of Medical Specialties or membership on the faculty of a Royal College. Two years of practice are required after completion of formal training in a medical or surgical specialty. No formal training in pain medicine is required. The examination is usually given in late winter (February) immediately after a review course given by the American Academy of Pain Medicine (AAPM). No recertification is currently required. Only one best answer questions appear on the examination; there are no K-type questions. The current content distribution is 20 percent anatomy and physiology, 20 percent types of pain, 20 percent pharmacology, 5 percent medical diagnostics, 10 percent pain assessment, 10 percent medical and surgical treatments, 10 percent psychiatric, and 5 percent compensation, disability, and rehabilitation medicine. Successful examinees become Diplomates of the American Board of Pain Medicine. For a full content outline and more information regarding this examination, contact the American Board of Pain Medicine, 5700 Old Orchard Road, Skokie, IL 60077. The phone number is (708) 966-9510 and the fax number is (708) 966-9418.

The American Academy of Pain Management (AAPM) offers the only examination available to pain practitioners who are not doctors of medicine or osteopathy. A medical license, formal training in pain, and certification by the American Board of Medical Specialties are *not* required. Two years of clinical experience working with patients with pain complaints is required. The yearly written examination consists of 100 questions. The current content distribution of the examination is 20 to 25 percent compensation, disability, and rehabilitation medicine; 20 to 25 percent psychiatric; 20 to 25 percent medical and surgical treatments; 5 to 10 percent pain assessment; 10 percent medical diagnostics; and 5 to 10 percent anatomy and physiology. Successful examinees will receive Diplomate, Fellow, Clinical Associate, Clinical Adjunct, or Affiliate status, depending on their level of higher education and pain management experience. For a full content outline and more information regarding this examination, contact the American Academy of Pain Management, 3600 Sisk Road, Suite 2D, Modesto, CA 95356. The phone number is (209) 545-0754 and the fax number is (209) 545-2920.

Various review courses are available to prepare for the examination. The Osler Review Course is a full 4-day course that intensively prepares the participant especially well for the ABA examination. The 3½-day PAINET review course has a broad focus that serves as very good preparation for the ABPM examination. Both review courses provide exposure to the wide range of topics covered on both examinations. The AAPM review course given just prior to the ABPM examination serves as an excellent general overview for the potential examinee as well as the experienced clinician. Because of the broad range of topics covered, as well as the detailed knowledge required to successfully complete the ABA and the ABPM examinations, we recommend that the review courses be used as supplements to intensive personal study rather than as your sole learning tool. Controversial topics are generally not covered on the examinations. Most questions address basic knowledge necessary for the successful practice of pain medicine. Review of a major text on pain medicine is also recommended prior to taking the examinations.

Good Luck!

Introduction

Each question is accompanied by an answer, a paragraph explanation, and a specific page reference to an appropriate textbook or journal article. A bibliography listing sources can be found following the last chapter of this text, and a list of abbreviations follows the introduction.

As you proceed, indicate your answer beside each question. After you finish going through the questions in each section, spend as much time as you need verifying your answers and carefully reading the explanations provided. Pay special attention to the explanations for the questions you answered incorrectly—but read *every* explanation. The authors of this material have designed the explanations to reinforce and supplement the information tested by the questions. If you feel you need further information about the material covered, you can consult and study the references indicated.

Abbreviations

AAG	Alpha 1-acid glycoprotein	**HTM**	High-threshold mechanoreceptor
ABI	Ankle brachial index	**IBQ**	Illness behavior questionnaire
ACTH	Adrenocorticotropic hormone	**mA**	Milliampere
AED	Antiepileptic drug	**MMPI**	Minnesota Multiphasic Personality Inventory
AHZ	Acute herpes zoster		
AIDS	Autoimmune deficiency syndrome	**MPQ**	McGill Pain Questionnaire
ALQ	Anterolateral quadrant	**MRI**	Magnetic resonance imaging
AV	Atrioventricular	**MS**	Multiple sclerosis
BOTOX	Botulinum toxin	**MSG**	Monosodium glutamate
CGRP	Calcitonin gene–related peptide	**NCS**	Nerve conduction study
CNS	Central nervous system	**NMDA**	N-methyl-D-aspartate
CPH	Chronic paroxysmal hemicrania	**PABA**	Para-aminobenzoic acid
C-PMN	C-polymodal nociceptor	**PAG**	Periaqueductal gray
CSF	Cerebrospinal fluid	**PCA**	Patient-controlled analgesia
CT	Computed tomography	**PT**	Prothrombin time
DADL	D-alanine, D-leucine	**PVG**	Periventricular gray
DREZ	Dorsal root entry zone	**PLL**	Posterior longitudinal ligament
ECG	Electrocardiogram	**RSD**	Reflex sympathetic dystrophy
EMG	Electromyogram	**SCI**	Spinal cord injury
ESR	Erythrocyte sedimentation rate	**SCS**	Spinal cord stimulation
GABA	Gamma-aminobutyric acid	**SEP**	Somatosensory evoked potential
GI	Gastrointestinal	**SHP**	Superior hypogastric plexus
5-HETE	5-Hydroxyeicosatetraenoic acid	**SLR**	Straight leg raise

ABBREVIATIONS

SMT	Spinomesencephalic tract	**TMJ**	Temporomandibular joint
SRT	Spinoreticular tract	**VIP**	Vasoactive intestinal polypeptide
SSRI	Selective serotonin reuptake inhibitor	**VPL**	Ventroposterolateral
STT	Spinothalamic tract	**VPM**	Ventroposteromedial
TCA	Tricyclic antidepressant	**WDR**	Wide dynamic range (neurons)
TENS	Transcutaneous electrical nerve stimulation		

Pain Management
PreTest® Self-Assessment and Review

Anatomy and Physiology

DIRECTIONS: Each question below contains suggested responses. Select the **one best** response.

1. All the following statements about the "wind-up" phenomenon are true EXCEPT

   (A) prolonged hyperexcitability of spinal dorsal horn neurons increases with repeated C-fiber input
   (B) the spinal cord neurons receive the C-fiber impulses and respond with greater discharges when input arrives at intervals of less than 3 s
   (C) wind-up does not play a role in the pain experienced by patients with reflex sympathetic dystrophy (RSD)
   (D) Mk-801 decreases Fos protein expression in the superficial laminae of the dorsal horn
   (E) the early immediate gene C-Fos activity increases after nerve injury to produce Fos protein within 2 h after nerve section

2. Regarding a myelinated nerve fiber, all the following statements are true EXCEPT

   (A) the action potential is regenerated only at the nodes of Ranvier
   (B) the resting potential is about −90 microvolts (μV)
   (C) sodium channels are present only at the nodes of Ranvier
   (D) potassium ions flow inward across the cell membrane during depolarization

3. Which Rexed lamina has the highest concentration of wide dynamic range neurons?

   (A) I
   (B) II
   (C) III
   (D) V
   (E) IX

4. Meckel's cave is

   (A) located between the mastoid process and the angle of the mandible
   (B) the recess in which the gasserian ganglion resides before dividing into the branches of the trigeminal nerve
   (C) an intestinal diverticulum that may cause epigastric pain
   (D) the location of the glossopharyngeal nerve as it passes near the tonsillar fossa
   (E) the retrouterine recess in which an abscess or tumor may compress the hypogastric plexus

5. A patient presents with a chief complaint of pain over and around a scar on the left thigh. On examination, there is an old, well-healed scar on the anterior aspect of the left thigh. The patient states that even light touch causes severe pain. Pinching the area is intolerable. Each of the following terms could describe this pain problem EXCEPT

   (A) primary hyperalgesia
   (B) secondary hyperalgesia
   (C) hyperpathia
   (D) allodynia
   (E) referred pain

6. All the following statements are true of spinal nerves EXCEPT

   (A) they exit the spinal canal at the intervertebral foramina
   (B) thoracic spinal nerves form the intercostal nerves
   (C) they are derived from ventral and dorsal roots of the spinal cord
   (D) the dorsal rami combine to form plexuses at the cervical and lumbosacral levels

7. Most A-delta and C fibers

   (A) are myelinated
   (B) end as free nerve endings
   (C) terminate in the deep dermis
   (D) end as specific nociceptive receptors
   (E) terminate in specialized structures

8. All the following have been identified as algogenic substances EXCEPT

   (A) serotonin
   (B) leukotrienes
   (C) G protein
   (D) acetylcholine
   (E) histamine

9. All the following tracts are primarily involved with transmission of sensation EXCEPT

   (A) spinocerebellar
   (B) fasciculus gracilis
   (C) spinothalamic
   (D) fasciculus cuneatus
   (E) corticospinal

10. Correct statements regarding the sympathetic nervous system include which of the following?

    (A) It has cell bodies of preganglionic neurons in the anterolateral quadrant of the spinal cord
    (B) It has axons that pass via posterior spinal roots to reach paravertebral ganglia
    (C) It has lumbar ganglia that lie on the posterolateral surface of the respective vertebrae
    (D) It has paravertebral ganglia that extend from the second cervical vertebra to the coccyx

11. A plexus differs from a ganglion in that

    (A) a plexus refers to prevertebral ganglia only
    (B) a plexus refers to a site of synaptic connections specific to the sympathetic system
    (C) a plexus may be either sympathetic or parasympathetic
    (D) a plexus refers to ganglia and axons (sympathetic and parasympathetic) in a defined anatomic location

12. Which of the following ganglia transmit purely sympathetic impulses?

    (A) Ciliary
    (B) Sphenopalatine
    (C) Otic
    (D) Stellate

13. Abdominal autonomic plexuses include all the following EXCEPT the

    (A) celiac plexus
    (B) inferior hypogastric plexus
    (C) superior hypogastric plexus
    (D) esophageal plexus

14. The cells of the adrenal medulla are homologous to

    (A) postganglionic parasympathetic neurons
    (B) preganglionic sympathetic neurons
    (C) cholinergic interneurons
    (D) preganglionic parasympathetic neurons
    (E) postganglionic sympathetic neurons

ANATOMY AND PHYSIOLOGY

15. All the following statements regarding partial agonists are true EXCEPT

    (A) the slope of the dose-response curve is less steep than that of a full agonist
    (B) the dose-response curve exhibits a ceiling effect
    (C) concomitant administration of a partial and a full agonist can antagonize the effect of the full agonist
    (D) the agent can act as an agonist at one receptor and an antagonist at another

16. What is the diameter and conduction velocity of the A-beta fibers, which transmit small motor, touch, and pressure impulses?

    (A) 20 microns (μ), 5 meters per second (m/s)
    (B) 20 μ, 100 m/s
    (C) 4 μ, 20 m/s
    (D) 4 μ, 5 m/s

17. The patellar reflex is innervated by

    (A) L2–L4
    (B) L1–L4
    (C) L3–L5
    (D) L2–L5

18. Which of the following reflexes has the same lumbar innervation as the patellar reflex?

    (A) Internal hamstring reflex
    (B) Adductor reflex
    (C) Tensor fascia lata reflex
    (D) External hamstring reflex

19. The Achilles tendon reflex is innervated by which nerve?

    (A) Saphenous
    (B) Femoral
    (C) Deep peroneal
    (D) Tibial

20. For optimal epidural analgesia after a hysterectomy, the epidural insertion site should be close to

    (A) T9–T10
    (B) L1–L2
    (C) L3–L4
    (D) L5–S1

21. All the following are true statements regarding the sacral canal EXCEPT

    (A) it contains the cauda equina
    (B) its inferior border is the sacral hiatus
    (C) it has a mean volume of 15 mL
    (D) it communicates laterally with the sacral foramina
    (E) it contains the filum terminale

22. The maxillary nerve leaves the cranial cavity by way of the

    (A) foramen ovale
    (B) foramen spinosum
    (C) foramen rotundum
    (D) jugular foramen
    (E) foramen lacerum

23. The mandibular nerve leaves the cranial cavity by way of the

    (A) foramen ovale
    (B) foramen spinosum
    (C) foramen rotundum
    (D) jugular foramen
    (E) foramen lacerum

24. Each of the following nerves passes in front of the ear to provide innervation of the scalp EXCEPT the

    (A) supratrochlear nerve
    (B) great auricular nerve
    (C) zygomaticotemporal nerve
    (D) supraorbital nerve
    (E) auriculotemporal nerve

25. The styloid process is an important landmark when one performs a blockade of the

    (A) phrenic nerve
    (B) maxillary nerve
    (C) facial nerve
    (D) glossopharyngeal nerve
    (E) trigeminal nerve

26. The recurrent laryngeal nerve supplies motor function to all the intrinsic muscles of the larynx EXCEPT the

    (A) sternothyroid
    (B) sternohyoid
    (C) thyrohyoid
    (D) cricoarytenoid
    (E) cricothyroid

27. A 36-year-old is undergoing a cervical plexus block for manipulation of a frozen shoulder. After the block is performed, it is noted that the patient is unable to elevate the shoulder. Which of the following nerves was blocked during the cervical plexus block?

    (A) Thoracodorsal
    (B) Accessory
    (C) Anterior cervical
    (D) Supraclavicular
    (E) Greater articular

28. Each of the following nerves is a branch of the maxillary nerve contained within the pterygopalatine fossa EXCEPT the

    (A) inferior alveolar
    (B) greater palatine
    (C) nasopalatine
    (D) superior alveolar
    (E) pharyngeal

29. The afferent limb of the oculocardiac reflex is by way of which nerve?

    (A) Facial
    (B) Optic
    (C) Ophthalmic
    (D) Vagus
    (E) Ciliary

30. The muscle involved in stabilizing the disk on the condyle of the temporomandibular joint (TMJ) is the

    (A) temporalis
    (B) buccinator
    (C) masseter
    (D) internal pterygoid
    (E) lateral pterygoid

31. The thorax of females differs from that of males in that

    (A) its capacity is greater
    (B) the cranial margin of the sternum is at the T2 level
    (C) its sternum is shorter
    (D) its upper ribs are less movable
    (E) it has a conical shape

32. When performing an epidural injection, each of the following structures is traversed EXCEPT the

    (A) supraspinous ligament
    (B) subcutaneous tissue
    (C) interspinous ligament
    (D) ligamentum flavum
    (E) posterior longitudinal ligament

33. The anterior surface of the head of each rib is connected to the sides of the bodies of two adjacent vertebrae by which ligament?

    (A) Intraarticular
    (B) Anterior longitudinal
    (C) Radiate
    (D) Superior costotransverse
    (E) Lateral costotransverse

34. The rib that articulates with the sternum at the level of the xiphisternal junction is the

    (A) 6th
    (B) 7th
    (C) 8th
    (D) 9th
    (E) 10th

35. The inner lining of the thoracic cage is also known as the

    (A) endothoracic fascia
    (B) external thoracic fascia
    (C) innermost intercostal muscles
    (D) visceral pleura
    (E) parietal pleura

36. The muscles that compose the anterior abdominal wall include all the following EXCEPT the

    (A) cremaster
    (B) internal oblique
    (C) transversus abdominis
    (D) iliacus
    (E) pyramidalis

37. The thoracic duct ascends from the abdominal cavity to enter the thorax via which aperture?

    (A) Esophageal
    (B) Central tendon
    (C) Splanchnic
    (D) Inferior vena caval
    (E) Aortic

38. All the following statements are true with regard to the superior hypogastric plexus EXCEPT that it

    (A) is located at the level of the aortic bifurcation
    (B) receives contributions from the L5 and S1 splanchnic nerves
    (C) often lies to the left of the midline
    (D) is a retroperitoneal structure
    (E) contains parasympathetic fibers derived from the pelvic splanchnic nerves

39. Characteristics of the lumbar vertebrae include

    (A) the body is wider anteroposteriorly than transversely
    (B) they are the smallest of the immovable vertebrae
    (C) the lumbar vertebral (spinal) canal is larger than the cervical canal
    (D) the lumbar vertebral (spinal) canal is larger than the thoracic canal

40. All the following are true statements concerning intervertebral disks EXCEPT

    (A) in the lumbar region, the disks constitute 30 percent of the length of the column
    (B) the nucleus pulposus is a colloidal gel composed of mucopolysaccharide
    (C) the annulus fibrosus is a fibrocartilaginous ring
    (D) the superior and inferior plates of the disk are composed of hyaline cartilage
    (E) at birth, an intervertebral disk contains 50 percent water

41. The posterior primary division of a spinal nerve provides sensory innervation to all the following structures EXCEPT

    (A) cutaneous and muscular structures
    (B) intervertebral (facet) joints
    (C) posterior ligaments
    (D) posterior longitudinal ligament
    (E) periosteum

42. Which of the following branches of the spinal artery provides blood supply to the vertebral body?

    (A) Anterior
    (B) Intermediate
    (C) Lateral
    (D) Medial
    (E) Posterior

43. Which of the following positions is associated with the greatest amount of load on the lumbar intervertebral disks?

    (A) Lying supine
    (B) Sitting, bending over
    (C) Sitting with back straight
    (D) Standing, flexed at the waist
    (E) Standing upright

44. All the following are true statements regarding pain and spinal cord lesions EXCEPT

    (A) both complete and incomplete spinal cord lesions can cause pain
    (B) the development of central pain after a spinal cord lesion depends on cord level
    (C) pain is usually produced in an area of somatosensory loss
    (D) spinal cord lesions commonly cause central pain
    (E) traumatic spinal cord lesions are the most common cause of central pain of spinal cord origin

45. The substantia gelatinosa resides in which laminar segment of the spinal cord?

    (A) I
    (B) II
    (C) V
    (D) VII
    (E) X

46. Muscle-stretch reflexes are diminished or absent in each of the following EXCEPT

(A) deep sedation
(B) strychnine poisoning
(C) deep coma
(D) nerve root block
(E) hypothyroidism

47. All the following statements regarding the *N*-methyl-D-aspartate (NMDA) receptor are true EXCEPT

(A) Mk-801 is a noncompetitive NMDA receptor antagonist
(B) NMDA may be involved in injury-induced wind-up
(C) glutamate and aspartate act at the NMDA receptor
(D) ketamine is an NMDA receptor agonist
(E) wind-up is prevented by NMDA antagonists

48. Each of the following is a function of the facial nerve EXCEPT

(A) it carries parasympathetic secretory fibers to the lacrimal glands
(B) it is involved in the afferent limb of the orbicularis oculi reflex
(C) it conveys taste sensation from the posterior two-thirds of the tongue
(D) it innervates muscles of facial expression
(E) it conveys exteroceptive sensation from the region of the eardrum

49. The intensity of a signal that is transmitted to the brain can be increased by increasing the frequency of impulses traveling along a single fiber. This is called

(A) spatial summation
(B) after-discharge
(C) temporal summation
(D) recruitment
(E) saltatory conduction

ANATOMY AND PHYSIOLOGY

DIRECTIONS: Each question below contains four suggested responses of which **one or more** is correct. Select

A	if	**1, 2, and 3**	are correct
B	if	**1 and 3**	are correct
C	if	**2 and 4**	are correct
D	if	**4**	is correct
E	if	**1, 2, 3, and 4**	are correct

50. Which of the following statements is true regarding the termination of the C-fiber primary afferents in the spinal cord?

    (1) C fibers enter mostly medial to the A-beta fibers in the dorsal root entry zone
    (2) C fibers collateralize into the tract of Lissauer
    (3) No C fibers exist within the ventral nerve roots
    (4) C fibers project rostrally and caudally in the tract of Lissauer

51. Statements that correctly describe mechanothermal nociceptors include

    (1) they are the most common type of nociceptor
    (2) they activate both A-delta and C fibers
    (3) they respond to both noxious mechanical and thermal stimuli
    (4) they may also be referred to as C-polymodal nociceptors

52. Visceral nociception is accurately characterized by which of the following statements?

    (1) It responds to cutting, burning, or crushing stimuli
    (2) It typically has a significant autonomic component
    (3) It involves more nociceptors than cutaneous nociception
    (4) It is often diffuse and poorly localized

53. Descending inhibitory pathways typically involve which of the following neurochemical mechanisms?

    (1) Noradrenergic
    (2) Enkephalinergic
    (3) Serotonergic
    (4) Cholinergic

54. Opiate receptors in the brainstem are found in the

    (1) nucleus raphe magnus
    (2) dorsal raphe nuclei
    (3) periaqueductal gray area
    (4) locus ceruleus

55. True statements regarding postoperative pain include

    (1) it is likely the result of somatic nociception
    (2) it is usually not of diagnostic importance
    (3) it does not prolong recovery from surgery
    (4) it has different psychological correlates than acute pain

56. Possible mechanisms for the production of neuropathic pain include

    (1) malfunction of the "gate"
    (2) generation of ectopic impulses by nerves
    (3) "crosstalk" between large and small fibers
    (4) malfunction of central processing

57. The pathophysiologic factors involved in neuropathic pain include

    (1) well-defined inhibitory mechanisms
    (2) poorly defined central pathways
    (3) well-defined nociceptive mechanisms
    (4) well-defined neurologic damage

SUMMARY OF DIRECTIONS

A	B	C	D	E
1,2,3 only	1,3 only	2,4 only	4 only	All are correct

58. Which of the following might be associated with sympathetic efferent overactivity?

    (1) Cutaneous nociceptive sensitivity
    (2) Alteration in piloerection
    (3) Alteration in blood flow to skin and muscle
    (4) Alteration of sweating

59. Physiologic processes involved in nociception include

    (1) transmission
    (2) modulation
    (3) perception
    (4) transduction

60. The central nervous system consists of

    (1) brain
    (2) cranial nerves
    (3) spinal cord
    (4) spinal nerves

61. Correct statements regarding cell bodies include that those

    (1) of somatic motor nerves lie in the anterior horn of the spinal cord
    (2) of cranial nerves lie in the sensory nuclei of the cranial nerve
    (3) of somatic sensory nerves lie in the dorsal root ganglia
    (4) of visceral sensory nerves lie in the autonomic nervous system

62. A-delta fibers can be characterized by which of the following statements?

    (1) They are myelinated
    (2) They do not respond to mechanical stimulation
    (3) They conduct impulses at a rate of 20 m/s
    (4) They are also called *low-threshold mechanoreceptors*

63. Sensitization of high-threshold mechanoreceptors

    (1) is associated with a higher threshold to thermal stimulation
    (2) requires repeated stimulation
    (3) is associated with a lower threshold to mechanical stimulation
    (4) results in increased frequency of discharge

64. True statements regarding C fibers include that they

    (1) are mostly nociceptive
    (2) respond to mechanical, thermal, and chemical stimuli
    (3) are unmyelinated
    (4) make up a small proportion of fibers in a peripheral nerve

65. C-polymodal nociceptors (C-PMNs)

    (1) have large receptive fields
    (2) do not undergo sensitization
    (3) are involved with secondary hyperalgesia
    (4) respond only to mechanical and thermal stimulation

66. Pain caused by a brief noxious stimulus and experienced as brief and sharp (first pain)

    (1) can be blocked by applying local anesthetic
    (2) can be blocked by applying pressure
    (3) is mediated by C-PMNs
    (4) can occur in response to a thermal stimulus

67. Which of the following will characteristically occur after injury to the skin?

    (1) Local edema
    (2) Intense vasoconstriction
    (3) Secondary vasodilation in adjacent areas
    (4) Increased threshold for nonnoxious stimuli

68. The sequence of events involved in neurogenic inflammation includes

    (1) spreading vasodilation
    (2) sensitization of C-PMNs
    (3) edema
    (4) secondary hyperalgesia

ANATOMY AND PHYSIOLOGY

69. Bradykinin, a peptide produced by activation of the kinin system,

(1) decreases vascular permeability
(2) has binding sites in the dorsal horn
(3) inhibits leukocyte chemotaxis
(4) is produced at sites of tissue injury

70. The class of compounds considered prostanoids includes

(1) prostacyclins
(2) thromboxanes
(3) prostaglandins
(4) leukotrienes

71. True statements regarding substance P include that it

(1) is synthesized in the dorsal root ganglia
(2) is released by stimulation of primary afferent nociceptors
(3) is transported to peripheral and central terminals
(4) inhibits the release of histamine

72. Administration of substance P causes which of the following?

(1) Plasma extravasation
(2) Pain on local injection
(3) Neurogenic inflammation
(4) Activation of nociceptors

73. Histamine is correctly described by which of the following?

(1) It causes edema
(2) It causes activation of nociceptors
(3) It causes vasodilation
(4) It is released from injured cells

74. True statements regarding serotonin include that it

(1) is an analgesic substance
(2) is released by platelets
(3) has no known antagonist
(4) has receptors located on peripheral nerves

75. Bone pain may be characterized by which of the following descriptions?

(1) It can originate from the cortex and marrow
(2) It is transmitted by A-delta and C fibers
(3) It has the highest pain threshold of the deep somatic structures
(4) It primarily arises from cancellous bone

76. Accurate descriptions of visceral afferent fibers include that they

(1) travel with sympathetic fibers
(2) are autonomic fibers
(3) have large receptive fields
(4) do not undergo sensitization

77. The brainstem is

(1) made up of the medulla, pons, and midbrain
(2) roofed by the fourth ventrical
(3) bounded rostrally by the thalamus
(4) bounded ventrally by the clivus

78. Criteria for neurotransmitters in primary afferent nociceptors include

(1) the substance is present in the dorsal horn synapse
(2) the substance is released on noxious stimulation
(3) release of the substance causes the same effect as stimulation of the primary afferent
(4) injection of the substance causes pain

79. Cells found in the dorsal horn include

(1) excitatory interneurons
(2) inhibitory interneurons
(3) projection cells
(4) wide dynamic range (WDR) neurons

80. Laminae I, II, and V in the dorsal horn

(1) project to the brainstem
(2) abolish cutaneous pain when cut
(3) produce analgesia when stimulated
(4) are major areas for convergence of nociceptive transmission

SUMMARY OF DIRECTIONS				
A	B	C	D	E
1,2,3 only	1,3 only	2,4 only	4 only	All are correct

81. Ascending nociceptive pathways in the anterolateral quadrant (ALQ) of the spinal cord include the

    (1) spinothalamic tract
    (2) spinomesencephalic tract
    (3) spinoreticular tract
    (4) spinomedullary system

82. The reticular formation is accurately described by which of the following statements?

    (1) It regulates motor, sensory, and autonomic functions
    (2) It consists of nuclei located in the brainstem
    (3) It responds to noxious stimulation
    (4) It is involved with the affective component of pain

83. True statements regarding serotonin include

    (1) it is found in the rostroventral medulla
    (2) it inhibits nociceptive neurons in laminae V and X
    (3) it is involved in descending antinociceptive pathways
    (4) its direct application to the spinal cord has no effect on pain

84. The major anatomic areas of the CNS involved in opioid-mediated analgesia include the

    (1) periventricular region
    (2) rostroventral medulla
    (3) periaqueductal gray matter
    (4) thalamus

85. The parasympathetic nervous system includes

    (1) axons that travel with the accessory nerve
    (2) cell bodies of preganglionic fibers in cranial nerve nuclei
    (3) short preganglionic fibers
    (4) cell bodies in the intermediolateral gray area of the sacral spinal cord

86. Acetylcholine is released at

    (1) preganglionic parasympathetic nerve endings
    (2) preganglionic sympathetic nerve endings
    (3) postganglionic parasympathetic nerve endings
    (4) postganglionic sympathetic nerve endings

87. Muscarinic receptors are located in all effector cells stimulated by

    (1) preganglionic sympathetic neurons
    (2) postganglionic parasympathetic neurons
    (3) preganglionic parasympathetic neurons
    (4) postganglionic cholinergic sympathetic neurons

88. Stimulation of which of the following receptors serves as a negative feedback mechanism?

    (1) Beta-1
    (2) Beta-2
    (3) Alpha-1
    (4) Alpha-2

89. Enkephalins are found in the

    (1) sympathetic nervous system
    (2) gastrointestinal tract
    (3) periaqueductal gray
    (4) adrenal medulla

90. Beta-endorphin is found in the

    (1) locus ceruleus
    (2) hypothalamus
    (3) periaqueductal gray
    (4) pituitary

91. Prototypic kappa-receptor agonists include

    (1) dynorphin
    (2) N-allyl normetazocine
    (3) ketocyclazocine
    (4) DADL

92. True statements regarding tolerance include

    (1) it is characteristic of opioids as a class of drugs
    (2) it cannot occur without physical dependence
    (3) it is defined as requiring more drug to produce the same effect
    (4) it is synonymous with addiction

93. Opioid peptides are derived from larger prohormones that include

    (1) proenkephalin A
    (2) proopiomelanocortin
    (3) proenkephalin B
    (4) alpha neoendorphin

94. True statements regarding alpha 1-acid glycoprotein include that it

    (1) has a high capacity
    (2) has a high affinity for basic drugs
    (3) remains unaffected by recent trauma
    (4) is an acute-phase reactant

95. Saltatory conduction is correctly described by which of the following?

    (1) It occurs in myelinated nerves
    (2) It occurs in unmyelinated nerves
    (3) It greatly increases the velocity of nerve conduction
    (4) It expends more energy

96. A neuron contains

    (1) a cell body
    (2) a dendrite
    (3) an axon
    (4) a synapse

97. Sensory receptors include

    (1) thermoreceptors
    (2) electromagnetic receptors
    (3) nociceptors
    (4) mechanoreceptors

98. Inhibitory neurotransmitters include

    (1) glycine
    (2) glutamic acid
    (3) gamma-aminobutyric acid (GABA)
    (4) substance P

99. Neuronal excitability is enhanced by

    (1) alkalosis
    (2) inhaled anesthetics
    (3) hyperventilation
    (4) hypoxemia

100. Withdrawal reflexes are correctly described by which of the following statements?

    (1) They are most often elicited by a stretch stimulus
    (2) They are transmitted by pathways that pass directly to anterior motor neurons
    (3) They typically take 1 to 2 s to occur
    (4) They are associated with extension of the opposite limb

101. Cranial tissues that are sensitive to pain include

    (1) pia mater
    (2) arteries of the dura mater
    (3) brain parenchyma
    (4) cranial sinuses and afferent veins

102. Receptor types that mediate analgesia include

    (1) delta
    (2) kappa
    (3) mu-1
    (4) mu-2

103. Changes that have been shown to take place after peripheral nerve injury include which of the following?

    (1) The primary afferent nerve endings in the spinal cord sprout new connections within the dorsal horn
    (2) Injured primary afferents may change neuropeptide production from substance P and calcitonin gene–related peptide (CGRP) to neuropeptide y, galanin, and vasoactive intestinal polypeptide (VIP)
    (3) Upregulation of C-Fos in intrinsic spinal neurons occurs
    (4) There is a large increase in the endogenous opioid dynorphin

SUMMARY OF DIRECTIONS

A	B	C	D	E
1,2,3 only	1,3 only	2,4 only	4 only	All are correct

104. Enkephalins are found in the
    (1) lungs
    (2) CNS
    (3) bladder
    (4) adrenal medulla

105. Nerve fibers primarily responsible for the transmission of pain impulses include
    (1) A-beta fibers
    (2) A-delta fibers
    (3) B fibers
    (4) C fibers

106. True statements regarding epidural veins include
    (1) they communicate with abdominal veins via the intervertebral foramina
    (2) they lie in the anterolateral part of the epidural space
    (3) they are large and valveless
    (4) they decrease in size if inferior vena caval obstruction is present

107. Landmarks used in performing a deep cervical plexus block include the
    (1) mastoid process
    (2) cricoid cartilage
    (3) Chassaignac's tubercle (C6)
    (4) posterior border of sternocleidomastoid muscle

108. The extraocular muscles innervated by CN III include the
    (1) lateral rectus
    (2) medial rectus
    (3) superior oblique
    (4) inferior rectus

109. The term *floating* applies to which ribs?
    (1) 1st
    (2) 11th
    (3) 2nd
    (4) 12th

110. True statements regarding the ligamentum flavum include
    (1) it is thinnest in the cervical region
    (2) it connects the laminae of adjacent vertebrae
    (3) it is thickest in the lumbar region
    (4) its fibers are arranged parallel to the laminae to which it is attached

111. The innervaton of the diaphagm includes
    (1) vagus nerves
    (2) intercostal nerves
    (3) lumbar plexus
    (4) cervical plexus

112. Except for the first intercostal nerve, all intercostal nerves differ from other spinal nerves in that
    (1) each pursues an independent course
    (2) they only have a sensory modality
    (3) they do not result in the formation of a plexus
    (4) their posterior divisions only supply muscles of the back

113. The visceral pleura receives innervation from
    (1) intercostal nerves
    (2) sympathetic fibers with vasomotor function
    (3) primary nociceptive afferent fibers
    (4) parasympathetic fibers via the pulmonary plexus

114. The abdominal wall is divided into nine imaginary quadrants, which include
    (1) left iliac
    (2) right hypochondriac
    (3) epigastric
    (4) hypergastric

115. True statements with regard to the celiac plexus include
    (1) it lies anterior to the crura of the diaphragm
    (2) the entire plexus lies posterior to the stomach and omental bursa
    (3) it is composed of parasympathetic and sympathetic fibers
    (4) it lies anterior to the vertebral body of L1

ANATOMY AND PHYSIOLOGY

116. True statements regarding the pudendal nerve include

    (1) it is derived from the S2, S3, and S4 nerves
    (2) it leaves the pelvic cavity through the greater sciatic foramen
    (3) it receives sympathetic fibers from the sacral portion of the sympathetic trunk
    (4) it divides into five main branches

117. Characteristics of the posterior longitudinal ligament (PLL) include that

    (1) it begins to progressively widen below the L1 vertebral level
    (2) it extends along the posterior surface of the body of the vertebra
    (3) it is composed of fibers that are less compact than those of the anterior longitudinal ligament
    (4) it contributes to the anterior wall of the vertebral canal

118. The intervertebral disk is correctly characterized by which of the following statements?

    (1) It receives blood supply from vessels in the bodies of adjacent vertebrae
    (2) It receives nutrients by diffusion after its blood supply diminishes
    (3) It receives nutrients by alternating compression and relaxation of the annulus fibrosus
    (4) It becomes avascular after the sixth decade of life

119. The posterior articulations, or facet joints, in the lumbar spine

    (1) permit rotation
    (2) comprise two arthrodial joints lined with synovium
    (3) allow lateral flexion or bending in the lordotic curve
    (4) lie in a vertical sagittal plane, permitting flexion and extension

120. True statements regarding the epidural space include that it is

    (1) bound anteriorly by the posterior longitudinal ligament
    (2) triangular in the lumbar region
    (3) bound posteriorly by the ligamentum flavum
    (4) most narrow anteriorly

121. Neuralgic pain differs from nociceptive pain in that it usually

    (1) has a delayed onset after a causative event
    (2) is responsive to opioid administration
    (3) has a dysesthetic component to it
    (4) can be treated by proximal surgical interruption

122. Exteroceptive sensations include

    (1) temperature
    (2) pain
    (3) touch
    (4) distention

123. Cranial nerves involved in the corneal reflex include

    (1) CN VII
    (2) CN III
    (3) CN V
    (4) CN VI

124. The cremaster reflex is correctly described by which of the following statements?

    (1) It is mediated through the ilioinguinal nerve
    (2) It is mediated through the genitofemoral nerve
    (3) It is evoked by stroking the inner thigh
    (4) It results in bilateral elevation of the testicles

Anatomy and Physiology

Answers

1. **The answer is C.** *(Ferrante, pp 47–48. Wall, pp 205–232.)* If a dorsal horn neuron is repetitively stimulated by a sufficient stimulus, it will activate C fibers and the frequency of discharge of the dorsal horn neuron will increase, as will pain perception. This phenomenon is called *cord wind-up*, or *central hypersensitization*. It can occur in the absence of sensitization of the peripheral nociceptors. Recent studies have shown that there is evidence of cord wind-up in some patients with RSD. Cord wind-up is more likely to occur when input arrives rapidly and continuously (at less than 3-s intervals). Within 2 h after nerve injury, the immediate early C-fos activity increases and there is upregulation of Fos protein production. Increase in Fos protein correlates with the presence of wind-up. Ketamine and Mk-801 can decrease Fos protein production and consequently decrease wind-up. *N*-methyl-D-aspartate (NMDA) receptor antagonists (ketamine and Mk-801) abolish central sensitization without altering the usual response of dorsal horn cells to painful stimuli.

2. **The answer is D.** *(Stoelting, pp 575–576. Raj, pp 137–138.)* An action potential occurs when an electrical, mechanical, or chemical stimulus increases neural membrane permeability to ion influx. The resting transmembrane potential is around $-90\ \mu V$ with high membrane permeability to potassium (K^+) and limited sodium (Na^+) permeability. As increasing stimuli alter the membrane potential, the membrane becomes much more permeable to Na^+. This causes sodium to flow in and potassium ions to flow outward. Chloride ion diffuses freely through the membrane in response to changes in polarity. The opening and closing of K^+ channels in response to stimuli is responsible for the depolarization and repolarization phases of the action potential. An ion channel, for example, enlarges during the depolarization phase ($+60$ to $70\ \mu V$). After depolarization, the Na^+ channels lose their increased permeability to Na^+, and K^+ is pumped back into the cells during repolarization. The potential gradually returns to resting transmembrane potential. The resting potential is maintained by diffusion of intracellular K^+ out of the cell through partially open K^+ channels. In myelinated nerves, the action potentials occur at the nodes of Ranvier and impulses are rapidly conducted by saltatory conduction. In nonmyelinated nerves, the action potentials occur along the length of the axon. Such continuous conduction is much slower than the saltatory conduction of myelinated fibers.

3. **The answer is D.** *(Wall, p 248.)* The Rexed laminae in the dorsal horn of the spinal cord are important in the modulation and transmission of nociceptive stimuli. Laminae I and II receive dense projections from the brainstem nuclei. Small diameter primary afferents also terminate primarily in laminae I and II. Myelinated primary afferent neurons and those from the brainstem involved in modulation of pain perception in laminae I and II also project to the deeper laminae such as V. Lamina V has a high concentration of wide dynamic range cells, which play an active role in the phenomenon of central sensitization.

4. **The answer is B.** *(Raj, p 713.)* The gasserian ganglion, also known as the trigeminal ganglion, is formed from many midpontine rootlets as they pass into the posterior cranial fossa and cross the superior border of the petrous bone to enter the recess called Meckel's cave, or the trigeminal cave. In this recess, the posterior two-

thirds of the ganglion are covered by dura. The anterior one-third is not covered by dura, and it is from this portion of the ganglion that the three major divisions of the trigeminal nerve (ophthalmic, maxillary, and mandibular) exit. When performing a trigeminal ganglion block, it is important to aspirate for blood and cerebrospinal fluid. If the needle has punctured the dura of Meckel's cave, a very small amount of local anesthetic may result in rapid loss of consciousness or cardiac arrest.

5. **The answer is E.** *(Raj, p 67.)* When the nociceptor is activated, functional changes occur. Tissue damage results in hyperalgesia both at the site of the injury (primary hyperalgesia) and in the surrounding area (secondary hyperalgesia). This results in a decrease in the pain threshold, with the potential for spontaneous pain, pain from normally nonnoxious stimuli (allodynia), and an exaggerated response to noxious stimuli (hyperpathia).

6. **The answer is D.** *(Ferrante, pp 18–19.)* Spinal nerves are derived from the union of the corresponding ventral and dorsal roots of the spinal cord. They exit the spinal canal through the intervertebral foramina and immediately split into dorsal and ventral rami. The dorsal rami pass posteriorly to innervate the paraspinal muscles and skin. The ventral rami combine to form plexuses at cervical and lumbosacral levels. The thoracic spinal nerves form the intercostal nerves.

7. **The answer is B.** *(Ferrante, pp 22–23.)* Most A-delta and C fibers do not terminate in specialized structures but end as free nerve endings. A-delta fibers terminate in the epidermis, while C fibers may end in the superficial dermis. Despite careful searches for a specific structure for a nociceptive receptor, it appears that transduction of noxious stimulation occurs in the free nerve ending.

8. **The answer is C.** *(Ferrante, pp 27, 641.)* Accumulation of algogenic substances in the area of injury is an integral part of the mechanism underlying transduction and sensitization. A number of such substances have been identified, including potassium, hydrogen ion, serotonin, histamine, bradykinin, acetylcholine, prostaglandins, leukotrienes, and substance P. The G protein (guanine nucleotide binding protein) promotes transmembrane signaling to a discrete effector mechanism, which may be a transmembrane ion channel or an intracellular second-messenger cascade.

9. **The answer is E.** *(Ferrante, p 33.)* The spinothalamic tract subserves the sensations of pain and temperature. Fibers associated with proprioception and crude touch enter the dorsal horn and ascend ipsilaterally in the dorsal columns (fasciculus gracilis and fasciculus cuneatus). Unconscious sensation is mediated by the spinocerebellar tract. The major descending tract is the corticospinal tract, which is responsible for motor activity.

10. **The answer is D.** *(Ferrante, p 72.)* Cell bodies of preganglionic sympathetic neurons lie within the intermediolateral gray of spinal cord segments T1–L2. Axons from these preganglionic neurons pass by way of anterior spinal roots and rami communicantes to reach paravertebral ganglia of the sympathetic chain. Paravertebral ganglia are segmentally arrayed in bilateral vertical rows extending from the second cervical vertebra to the coccyx. Lumbar ganglia lie on the anterolateral surface of the respective vertebrae.

11. **The answer is D.** *(Ferrante, p 73.)* A ganglion refers to a site of synaptic connections specific to the sympathetic or parasympathetic systems. Plexus refers to a number of ganglia and axons (sympathetic and parasympathetic, as well as visceral afferent) converging in a well-defined anatomic location.

12. **The answer is D.** *(Ferrante, p 73.)* Autonomic ganglia include the ciliary, sphenopalatine, otic, and submaxillary ganglia, which are situated in relation to the respective cranial nerves (III, VII, and IX). Each ganglion receives sympathetic postganglionic fibers, parasympathetic preganglionic fibers, and sensory fibers. The superior, middle, intermediate, and inferior ganglia compose the sympathetic chain within the cervical region. The stellate ganglion is another term for the inferior cervical ganglion, which lies behind the subclavian artery, near the origin of the vertebral artery at the level of the seventh cervical vertebra. It is sometimes fused with the first thoracic ganglion.

13. **The answer is D.** *(Ferrante, p 74.)* The abdomen contains three large plexuses composed of prevertebral sympathetic ganglia, parasympathetic fibers from the vagus or sacral parasympathetics, and visceral afferent fibers. The celiac plexus innervates the abdominal viscera. The other two great abdominal plexuses include the superior and inferior hypogastric plexuses supplying the pelvic viscera.

14. **The answer is E.** *(Ferrante, p 76.)* Norepinephrine is the neurotransmitter found in postganglionic sympathetic (adrenergic) nerve endings. The cells of the adrenal medulla are homologous to postganglionic sympathetic neurons and contain both epinephrine (80 percent) and norepinephrine (20 percent).

15. **The answer is D.** *(Ferrante, pp 153–154.)* Partial agonists exhibit certain characteristic pharmacologic properties: (1) the slope of the dose-response curve is less steep than that of a full agonist; (2) the dose-response curve exhibits a ceiling effect (i.e., a submaximal response as compared with that of a full agonist); and (3) concomitant administration of a partial and a full agonist can reduce (antagonize) the effect of the full agonist. Mixed agonist-antagonists act simultaneously as an agonist at one receptor and an antagonist at another.

16. **The answer is B.** *(Ramamurthy, p 20.)* A-alpha, -beta, and -gamma myelinated fibers are 20 µ in diameter. They have a conduction velocity of 100 m/s. A-alpha fibers provide large motor function and proprioception and are responsible for reflex activity. A-beta fibers are responsible for small motor function, touch, and pressure. A-gamma fibers provide muscle tone via innervation of the muscle spindle fibers. A-delta fibers are myelinated fibers of 4 µ in diameter that conduct impulses at 5 m/s. They transmit temperature sensation, sharp pain, and possibly touch. C fibers are unmyelinated fibers of 0.5 to 1.0 µ with a conduction velocity of 1.2 m/s. They transmit dull pain, temperature, and touch.

17. **The answer is A.** *(Raj, p 104.)* The patellar (quadriceps) reflex is innervated by the femoral nerve (L2–L4). It is demonstrated by contraction of the quadriceps femoris muscle when the patellar tendon is tapped.

18. **The answer is B.** *(Raj, p 104.)* The adductor (tibioadductor) reflex is tested by tapping the medial epicondyle of the femur or the medial condyle of the tibia. The adductor muscle contracts, with inward movement of the thigh. The reflex is innervated by the obturator nerve (L2–L4). The patellar reflex is innervated by the femoral nerve (L2–L4). The internal hamstring reflex is supplied by L4–S2, the tensor fascia lata reflex by L4–L5, and the external hamstring reflex by L5–S2 or S3.

19. **The answer is D.** *(Raj, p 106.)* The Achilles tendon reflex is innervated by the tibial nerve (S1 and S2, possibly L5). The ankle jerk is often diminished when an S1 nerve root is affected. The saphenous nerve is L3–L4, the femoral nerve is L2–L4, and the deep peroneal nerve is L4–L5.

20. **The answer is A.** *(Bonica, p 135.)* To provide optimal analgesia using the least amount of local anesthetic after lower abdominal or pelvic surgery, the epidural catheter should be placed near the spinal cord segments that innervate the incision, *not* at the level at which the nerve roots exit. The spinal cord ends at about L2. The lumbar and sacral nerve roots must travel from their origin in the cord at the lower thoracic and upper lumbar levels to exit the lumbar and sacral foramina below.

21. **The answer is C.** *(Cousins, pp 365–366.)* The sacral canal is the continuation of the lumbar spinal canal. It communicates laterally with the anterior and posterior sacral foramina. Inferiorly, it terminates at the sacral hiatus. The volume of the sacral canal, including the sacral foraminal extensions, varies between 12 and 65 mL with a mean of about 30 to 34 mL. The canal contains the five sacral nerve roots and the coccygeal nerve, which constitute the cauda equina. Also found in the canal is the filum terminale, which exits through the sacral hiatus to attach to the back of the coccyx.

22. **The answer is C.** *(Cousins, p 534.)* The maxillary nerve leaves the cranial cavity by way of the foramen rotundum. From here it traverses the pterygomaxillary fossa to enter the floor of the orbit at the inferior orbital fissure. The maxillary nerve primarily supplies the upper jaw, lateral nasal wall, and most of the nasal septum.

ANATOMY AND PHYSIOLOGY ANSWERS

23. **The answer is A.** *(Cousins, p 534.)* The mandibular nerve emerges from the cranial cavity by way of the foramen ovale to enter the infratemporal fossa. In the infratemporal fossa the mandibular nerve divides into its terminal branches, which innervate the lower jaw, tongue, and lower teeth, the buccal surface of the cheek, and the skin overlying the lower jaw, the temporal region, and the anterosuperior two-thirds of the surface of the external ear.

24. **The answer is B.** *(Cousins, p 538.)* In the region of the scalp, there are eight nerves involved in processing sensory information. Four sensory nerves pass in front of the ear to the scalp: the supratrochlear and supraorbital nerves from V1 (trigeminal branch); the zygomaticotemporal nerve from V2 (trigeminal branch); and the auriculotemporal nerve from V3 (trigeminal branch). Four nerves pass behind the ear: the great auricular nerve and the greater, lesser, and least occipital nerves from the cervical plexus. All eight nerves converge toward the vertex of the scalp.

25. **The answer is D.** *(Cousins, p 540.)* The tip of the styloid process lies approximately halfway between the angle of the mandible and the mastoid process and provides a bony landmark for blockade of the glossopharyngeal nerve. The glossopharyngeal nerve exits the jugular foramen at the base of the skull to emerge slightly posterior and medial to the styloid process. It proceeds inferiorly to innervate the posterior one-third of the tongue as well as parts of the throat and nasopharynx as far down as the pharyngoesophageal junction at the level of the cricoid cartilage.

26. **The answer is E.** *(Cousins, p 540.)* Below the level of the vocal cords the larynx and trachea are innervated by the recurrent laryngeal branch of the vagus nerve. The recurrent laryngeal nerve not only provides sensation to the structures below the level of the cords, it also supplies motor function to all the intrinsic muscles of the larynx except the cricothyroid muscle. Bilateral blockade of the recurrent laryngeal nerve will result in loss of phonation as well as an inability to close the glottis.

27. **The answer is B.** *(Cousins, pp 545–551.)* Blockade of the accessory nerve (CN XI) is useful for trapezius muscle block as an adjunct to interscalene nerve blocks of the brachial plexus for surgery on the shoulder. The accessory nerve traverses the posterior triangle of the neck in a very superficial location. It emerges from the body of the sternocleidomastoid muscle at the junction of the superior and middle third of the posterior border of the muscle and therefore is frequently unintentionally blocked when a superficial cervical plexus block is performed.

28. **The answer is A.** *(Cousins, pp 566–572.)* Branches of the maxillary nerve within the pterygopalatine fossa include the pharyngeal branch to the mucosa of the pharynx, the greater palatine branch to the mucosa of the posterior palate, the nasopalatine branch to the septal mucosa through the incisive canal to the anterior hard palate, and the superior alveolar branch to the second and third maxillary molars. The inferior alveolar nerve is a sensory branch of the mandibular nerve that supplies the mandibular teeth, body of the mandible, and labial gingiva anterior to the bicuspid teeth.

29. **The answer is C.** *(Cousins, p 589.)* The oculocardiac reflex is defined as a slowing of the pulse in response to traction on the extraocular muscles or from pressure on the eye. The afferent arc is by way of the ophthalmic branch of the trigeminal nerve. Impulses travel through the reticular network to the visceral motor nuclei of the vagus nerve, which is the efferent limb of the reflex to the heart.

30. **The answer is E.** *(Raj, p 227.)* The lateral pterygoid muscle attaches anteriorly to the disk and condyle of the temporomandibular joint as the mouth is closed. The main muscles of jaw closure are the masseter, internal pterygoid, and temporalis muscles and the superior belly of the lateral pterygoid muscle.

31. **The answer is C.** *(Bonica, p 959.)* The female thorax differs from that of the male in several respects: the capacity of the female thorax is less; the sternum is shorter; and the cranial margin of the sternum is on a level with the caudal part of the body of the T3 vertebra, whereas in the male it is on a level with the caudal part of

the body of the T2 vertebra. Also, the upper ribs are more movable in the female thorax, permitting a greater expansion of the cranial part of the thorax. Both the male and female thoraces are conical in shape because the superior, or cervical, inlet is of a lesser diameter than the inferior abdominal part.

32. **The answer is E.** *(Bonica, p 962.)* When performing an epidural injection, the needle must first enter skin and subcutaneous tissue with continued forward advancement. The supraspinous ligament, interspinous ligament, and ligamentum flavum are traversed, after which continued advancement places the needle in the epidural space. The supraspinous ligament is a strong, fibrous cord that connects the spinous processes from the C7 vertebra to the sacrum. The interspinous ligaments are thin and membranous and connect adjoining spinous processes, extending from the root to the apex of each process. The ligamenta flava connect the laminae of adjacent vertebrae, while the posterior longitudinal ligament extends from the axis to the sacrum and passes over the dorsal surface of the bodies of the vertebrae and the intervertebral disks. Although the posterior longitudinal ligament is the anterior boundary for the epidural space, it is not traversed when an epidural injection is performed.

33. **The answer is C.** *(Bonica, pp 962–963.)* The radiate ligament connects the anterior part of the head of each rib with the sides of the bodies of two adjacent vertebrae and the intervertebral disks between them. The intraarticular ligament consists of a short flat band of fibers attached at one end to the crest separating the two articular facets on the head of the rib and at the other end to the intervertebral disk. The superior costotransverse ligament is attached to the superior border of the neck of the rib and passes laterally to the lower border of the neck of the transverse process immediately above. The lateral costotransverse ligament passes from the apex of the transverse process of the vertebra to the rough and nonarticular portion of the tubercle of the corresponding rib.

34. **The answer is B.** *(Bonica, p 963.)* The 7th costal cartilage articulates with the sternum at the lateral margin of the xiphisternal junction. The articulation between the xiphoid process and the inferior border of the sternal body is a cartilaginous structure that ossifies later in life. The joint is secured laterally by radiating fibers of the sternocostal ligaments.

35. **The answer is A.** *(Bonica, p 964.)* The rib cage is covered both internally and externally by thin layers of deep fascia. The inner layer, consisting of loose areolar tissue called the *endothoracic fascia*, lines the internal aspect of the thoracic cage. This layer of facia covers the inner surface of the intercostal muscles and intervening ribs, along with the subcostal and transversus thoracis muscles and the diaphragm. It lies between the parietal pleura and the thoracic cage.

36. **The answer is D.** *(Bonica, p 1150.)* The muscles of the abdomen are divided into an anterolateral group and a posterior group. The anterolateral group is composed of four flat muscular sheets that form the anterior abdominal wall. These muscles include the internal and external obliques; the transversus and rectus abdominis; and the cremaster and pyramidalis muscles, which are involved in suspending the testes and tensing the midline tendinous raphe of the abdominal wall, respectively. The iliacus is a posterior muscle of the abdominal wall.

37. **The answer is E.** *(Bonica, p 1150.)* The diaphragm has three large openings (the aortic, esophageal, and vena caval apertures) and a number of smaller ones that transmit the superior and middle splanchnic nerves. The aortic aperture is the lowest and most posterior of the large openings and approximates the level of the T10 vertebra. In addition to being an opening for the passage of the aorta, this aperture also transmits the thoracic duct and occasionally the azygous and hemiazygous veins.

38. **The answer is B.** *(Bonica, p 1290.)* The superior hypogastric plexus (SHP) is formed by the union of branches from the aortic plexus with contributions by the L3 and L4 splanchnic nerves. The plexus is situated in front of the bifurcation of the abdominal aorta, the body of the last lumbar vertebra, and the promontory of

the sacrum. It lies in the extraperitoneal connective tissue, often to the left of the midline. In addition to the sympathetic fibers that descend to form the SHP, the SHP contains parasympathetic fibers derived from the pelvic splanchnic nerves, which ascend from the inferior hypogastric plexus.

39. **The answer is D.** *(Bonica, p 1395.)* The lumbar vertebrae are the largest of the true immovable vertebrae and are also large in comparison to their own vertebral canal. The laminae are broad, short, and strong. The lumbar vertebral (spinal) canal is triangular and is larger than the thoracic canal but smaller than the cervical canal. The body of the vertebra is large and is wider transversely than anteroposteriorly and a little thicker anteriorly than posteriorly.

40. **The answer is E.** *(Bonica, p 1399.)* Each intervertebral disk is composed of a tough fibrocartilaginous ring (the annulus fibrosus) and a pliable intergelatinous mass (the nucleus pulposus). The colloidal gel of the nucleus pulposus is a mucopolysaccharide that can imbibe external fluid and maintain its intrinsic water balance. At birth the disk contains 88 percent water, but it dehydrates with age and trauma. In the lumbar region the intervertebral disks constitute about 30 percent of the length of the column as compared with 20 to 25 percent in the thoracic and cervical regions. The superior and inferior plates of the disk are the end plates of the vertebral bodies, which are composed of articular hyaline cartilage in direct contact with and adherent to the underlying resilient bone of the vertebral body.

41. **The answer is D.** *(Bonica, p 1401.)* In addition to the cutaneous and muscular distributions, the posterior primary division provides sensory fibers to fascia, ligaments, periosteum, and intervertebral (facet) joints. The meningeal nerves, also called the *sinovertebral*, or *recurrent*, *nerves of Luschka*, supply many structures within the spinal canal and also the longitudinal ligaments.

42. **The answer is A.** *(Bonica, p 1403.)* The spinal artery arises from the posterior branch of the segmental artery close to the intervertebral foramen and divides into three terminal branches: posterior, intermediate, and anterior. The posterior branches help supply the spinal dura and the tissues of the epidural space. The intermediate (middle) branches supply the dura of the associated nerve roots. Their radicular branch can pierce the dura and help supply the spinal cord. The anterior branches supply the vertebral bodies along with other spinal structures.

43. **The answer is B.** *(Bonica, p 1407.)* Relative loads on the L3 disk for various body positions compared with upright standing have been studied. With the subject lying, the load decreases significantly. Upright standing is equal to 100 percent of the relative load. In the sitting position with the back straight, the load is increased 40 percent above relaxed standing. With the subject standing and bending, the load increases 50 percent. With the patient sitting with the back unsupported or sitting and bending over, the load shows an even greater increase.

44. **The answer is B.** *(Bonica, p 266.)* Central pain of spinal cord origin most commonly occurs after traumatic spinal cord lesions. Spinal cord lesions of any cause commonly result in central pain. The pain usually occurs in an area of spinothalamic somatosensory loss. However, it may also occur with lesions that fail to produce clinically detectable somatosensory loss. Both complete and incomplete lesions, regardless of cord level, can cause central pain.

45. **The answer is B.** *(Bonica, p 41.)* Using cytoarchitectonic studies, Rexed divided the spinal gray into ten laminae, a classification that is now widely accepted. Laminae I through VI make up the dorsal horn, laminae VII through IX the ventral horn, and lamina X is composed of a column of cells clustered around the central canal of the cord. Lamina I is the marginal layer, lamina II is the substantia gelatinosa, and laminae II through V make up the nucleus propius (magnocellular layer).

46. The answer is B. *(Raj, pp 106–107.)* Diminution of the reflexes usually results from an interference with the conduction of an impulse through the reflex arc. Absence indicates a break in the reflex arc. The muscle-stretch reflexes may be either diminished or absent in deep coma, narcosis, deep sedation, and often in deep sleep. Reflexes are characteristically lost with nerve block, nerve root block, and caudal and spinal anesthesia. Hypothyroidism and severe toxemias also result in diminished or lost reflexes. Muscle-stretch reflexes are typically increased with pyramidal system lesions, early stages of coma and anesthesia, tetany, tetanus, and strychnine poisoning.

47. The answer is D. *(Wall, pp 233–234.)* NMDA receptors are involved in the activation of nociceptive neurons. The action of excitatory amino acids such as glutamate and aspartate at the NMDA receptor in the dorsal horn is enhanced by the neuropeptides substance P, calcitonin gene–related peptide (CGRP), and dynorphins. The corelease of excitatory amino acids and neuropeptides strengthens the synaptic connections in the dorsal horn and may increase the development of dorsal-horn hyperexcitability (cord wind-up). There is an expansion of the receptive fields of the wide dynamic range (WDR) neurons. Wind-up is prevented by NMDA receptor antagonists. Both Mk-801 and ketamine are NMDA receptor antagonists.

48. The answer is C. *(Raj, pp 90–91.)* Predominantly a motor nerve, the facial nerve innervates the muscles of facial expression. In addition, it carries parasympathetic secretory fibers to the salivary and lacrimal glands and to the mucous membranes of the oral and nasal cavities. It also conveys various types of sensation, including exteroceptive sensation from the region of the ear drum, taste sensation from the anterior two-thirds of the tongue, and general visceral sensation from the salivary glands and mucosa of the nose and pharynx. The facial nerve also contributes to the afferent limb of the orbicularis oculi reflex in conjunction with the trigeminal nerve.

49. The answer is C. *(Stoelting, pp 599–600.)* The overall pattern of several impulses relaying similar information is termed a *signal*. The intensity of a signal (such as pain) that is transmitted to the brain can be increased by increasing the number of parallel fibers participating (spatial summation) or by increasing the frequency of impulses traveling along a single fiber (temporal summation). The increase in the number of participating fibers as the intensity of a signal increases is termed *recruitment*. After-discharge is production of output signals for prolonged periods by a single input stimulus, and saltatory conduction is the process of successive excitation of nodes of Ranvier by an impulse that jumps between successive nodes.

50. The answer is C (2,4). *(Wall, pp 1057–1058.)* As small afferent axons (C and A-delta) enter the spinal cord, they are displaced *lateral* to the A-beta fibers (from muscle spindles and proprioceptive afferents) and trifurcate in the tract of Lissauer at the level of entry and with projections rostrally and caudally. Unmyelinated C fibers arising from the dorsal root ganglion cells also send projections into the ventral roots, which accounts for pain sensation that can occur with ventral root stimulation.

51. The answer is E (all). *(Raj, p 66.)* Modality-specific (e.g., heat) nociceptors exist, but the majority appear to respond to more than one noxious stimulus. The most common nociceptor appears to be the cutaneous mechanothermal nociceptor, which responds to noxious mechanical and thermal stimuli. Cutaneous mechanothermal nociceptors activate both A-delta and C fibers. The most common nociceptor in humans appears to be the C-fiber mechanothermal nociceptor, which responds to mechanical, thermal, and chemical stimuli.

52. The answer is C (2,4). *(Raj, p 67.)* There are significant clinical differences between visceral and cutaneous nociception. There are relatively fewer nociceptors in the viscera than in the skin, and these receptors may have a different activation profile. Cutting and burning mesentery, uterine cervix, or other organs does not necessarily produce clinical "pain," but traction, distention, or ischemia will produce pain. This pain is often diffuse and poorly localized and often has a significant autonomic component.

53. The answer is A (1,2,3). *(Raj, p 69.)* Centrifugal control of nociceptive transmission through the dorsal horn arises from a variety of structures that project descending inhibitory pathways. The pathways descending from these areas primarily involve noradrenergic, serotonergic, and enkephalinergic mechanisms. However, other mechanisms might also be involved.

54. The answer is A (1,2,3). *(Raj, p 71.)* The systemic administration of narcotic analgesics results in their binding to the specific opioid receptors in the cortex, brainstem, and spinal cord. The analgesic effect is in large part mediated by activation of descending control systems that originate in the brainstem. These brainstem areas, which include the periaqueductal gray area, the nucleus raphe magnus, and the dorsal raphe nuclei, are rich in opiate receptors. The locus ceruleus contains catecholamines, practically all of which are norepinephrine.

55. The answer is C (2,4). *(Raj, p 72.)* There are significant clinical differences between acute and postoperative pains. Postoperative pain is usually not of diagnostic importance, as the proximate cause of the pain is obvious tissue damage resulting from surgical trauma. It has been clearly shown that adequate relief of postoperative pain reduces both the morbidity and mortality of surgery and leads to earlier recovery from surgery. Postoperative pain has different psychological correlates than acute pain. It is likely to be a combination of somatic and visceral nociception.

56. The answer is E (all). *(Raj, p 73.)* There are four possible mechanisms for the production of pain in peripheral nerve lesions, as proposed by Wall: (1) the "gate" might be caused to malfunction, (2) the nerves might become mechanically sensitive and generate ectopic impulses, (3) there might be "crosstalk" between large and small fibers, and (4) there might be changes in the central processing.

57. The answer is C (2,4). *(Raj, p 74.)* Neuropathic pain is typically not biologically useful, although the neurologic damage may be well defined. Its nociceptive mechanisms, central pathways, and inhibitory mechanisms are poorly defined. Pain is often appreciated in a region of sensory deficit.

58. The answer is E (all). *(Raj, p 73.)* Pain following peripheral nerve damage has long been recognized as having a sympathetic component. It is clear that sympathetic afferents can transmit information of a nociceptive nature. However, one of the characteristics of this pain is that it is accompanied by sympathetic efferent overactivity. This may be reflected in alterations in the control of blood flow to the skin, muscles, and bone in the affected area and alterations in piloerection, sweating, and possibly cutaneous nociceptive sensitivity.

59. The answer is E (all). *(Ferrante, p 17.)* Nociception involves four physiologic processes. Transduction is the process whereby noxious stimuli are translated into electrical activity at the sensory endings of nerves. Transmission is the propagation of impulses throughout the sensory nervous system. Modulation is the process whereby nociceptive transmission is modified through a number of neural influences, and perception is the final process in which all aspects of pain are experienced.

60. The answer is B (1,3). *(Ferrante, p 18.)* The central nervous system consists of the brain and the spinal cord. The peripheral nervous system consists of the cranial and spinal nerves and their subsequent ramifications.

61. The answer is B (1,3). *(Ferrante, p 19.)* Cell bodies of somatic motor nerves lie in the anterior horn of the spinal cord or in motor nuclei of cranial nerves. Those of somatic sensory neurons reside in dorsal root ganglia, which are located in the intervertebral foramina. Sensory nerves subserving visceral sensation also have their cell bodies in dorsal root ganglia, though their axonal processes may travel with autonomic nerves to the periphery.

62. The answer is B (1,3). *(Ferrante, p 23.)* Myelinated fibers activated by noxious stimuli generally conduct in the A-delta range, about 20 m/s. They respond to mechanical stimulation. Although not as sensitive as large myelinated A-alpha fibers (so-called low-threshold mechanoreceptors), A-delta fibers dramatically increase their firing rate as the stimulus intensity becomes greater. Thus A-delta fibers are called *high-threshold mechanoreceptors*.

63. The answer is C (2,4). *(Ferrante, p 25.)* High-threshold mechanoreceptors (HTMs) do not fire in response to thermal stimulation unless stimuli are applied repeatedly. After repeated thermal stimulation, HTMs will become more sensitive (achieve a lower threshold to thermal stimulation) and will increase their frequency of discharge. This process is known as sensitization. The threshold for mechanical stimulation is unchanged by this process.

64. The answer is A (1,2,3). *(Ferrante, p 25.)* A large proportion of fibers in a peripheral nerve are C fibers. Most, if not all, of these fibers are nociceptive. Most C fibers respond to noxious mechanical, thermal, and chemical stimuli and are called C-polymodal nociceptors (C-PMNs).

65. The answer is B (1,3). *(Ferrante, pp 25–26.)* The receptive field for a C-PMN may be quite large (up to 17 mm^2). C-PMNs become sensitized after repeated noxious stimulation and may develop an ongoing discharge. Secondary hyperalgesia depends on activity in unmyelinated primary afferents with sensitization of C-PMNs.

66. The answer is C (2,4). *(Ferrante, p 26.)* Studies have shown that application of a brief noxious stimulus will initially be experienced as a brief, sharp pain (first pain). A more prolonged, dull sensation (second pain) follows after a short lull. Application of pressure will block first pain; application of local anesthetics will block second pain. First pain can occur in response to a thermal stimulus and is preferentially blocked by pressure. It is mediated by the A-delta mechanothermal nociceptor.

67. The answer is B (1,3). *(Ferrante, p 26.)* The characteristic sequence of events following a skin injury is known as the *triple response*: (1) intense vasodilation, (2) local edema (wheal), and (3) secondary vasodilation spreading to adjacent regions (flare). The subject will also note a decreased threshold to noxious stimuli and increased pain in response to noxious stimulation (primary hyperalgesia) in the injured area.

68. The answer is E (all). *(Ferrante, p 26.)* Secondary hyperalgesia depends on activity in unmyelinated primary afferents with sensitization of C-PMNs. After injury just outside their receptive fields, C-PMNs become sensitized and develop spontaneous depolarization. This activity of C-PMNs in areas of undamaged tissue causes spreading vasodilation, edema, and further sensitization of other C-PMNs within adjacent receptive fields. This sequence of events has been termed *neurogenic inflammation* because of its similarity to the inflammatory process.

69. The answer is C (2,4). *(Ferrante, p 27.)* Bradykinin is a 9–amino acid peptide produced at sites of tissue injury by enzymatic action. It produces pain in humans at concentrations equivalent to those found in injured tissue. Binding sites for bradykinin are found on sensory fibers and in the dorsal horn. Bradykinin also increases vascular permeability, enhances leukocyte chemotaxis, and sensitizes nociceptors.

70. The answer is A (1,2,3). *(Ferrante, p 27.)* Classes of compounds that appear in areas of tissue damage include the prostanoids and the eicosanoids. The prostanoids are the arachidonic acid metabolites of the cyclooxygenase pathway that comprise the thromboxanes, prostacyclins, and prostaglandins. The eicosanoids are the arachidonic acid metabolites of the lipoxygenase pathway including 5-hydroxyeicosatetraenoic acid (5-HETE) and the leukotrienes.

71. The answer is A (1,2,3). *(Ferrante, p 28.)* Substance P is an 11–amino acid peptide that was first identified in 1931 and later found to be associated with sensory transmission and vasodilation. Substance P is synthesized in the neuronal cell bodies in the dorsal root ganglia and transported to peripheral and central terminals, where it is stored in vesicles. It is released on stimulation of primary afferent nociceptors and causes vasodilation and edema. Substance P also causes release of histamine from mast cells, resulting in further vasodilation and edema.

ANATOMY AND PHYSIOLOGY ANSWERS

72. The answer is B (1,3). *(Ferrante, p 28.)* Administration of substance P provokes plasma extravasation; other peptides do not produce extravasation. However, despite its role in the initiation and augmentation of neurogenic inflammation, substance P does not produce pain on local injection nor does it activate nociceptors.

73. The answer is E (all). *(Ferrante, p 28.)* Histamine is released from injured cells and from mast cells stimulated by substance P. It causes activation of nociceptors, vasodilation, and edema.

74. The answer is C (2,4). *(Ferrante, p 28.)* Serotonin has been implicated as an algogenic substance. It is released by platelets in response to platelet-activating factor, a substance released by degranulating mast cells. Serotonin causes pain directly and by potentiation of the nociceptive effect of bradykinin. Its receptors are found on peripheral nerves, and antagonists will block the nociceptive effects of serotonin.

75. The answer is C (2,4). *(Ferrante, p 30.)* Bone is innervated by A-delta and C fibers that form a plexus around the periosteum and invest the cancellous bone. The cortex and marrow do not receive nociceptive fibers. Bone is said to have the lowest pain threshold of the deep somatic structures.

76. The answer is B (1,3). *(Ferrante, p 31.)* Visceral afferents generally travel with sympathetic fibers. They are not, however, autonomic fibers. Visceral afferents generally have large, confluent receptive fields and can be sensitized in response to certain conditions (inflammation).

77. The answer is E (all). *(Ferrante, pp 34–35.)* The brainstem is the most caudal portion of the brain and consists of the medulla (myelencephalon), pons (metencephalon), and midbrain (mesencephalon). It is bounded rostrally by the thalamus, caudally by the spinal cord, ventrally by a flat bone called the *clivus*, and dorsally by the fourth ventricle and cerebellum.

78. The answer is A (1,2,3). *(Ferrante, pp 44–45.)* Criteria for proving that a substance is a neurotransmitter for a primary afferent nociceptor are (1) presence of the substance in the dorsal horn synapse of the primary afferent, (2) release of the substance on noxious stimulation, (3) the same effect by release of the substance and stimulation of the primary afferent, and (4) blockade of the effect of both the substance and the primary afferent by administration of an antagonist.

79. The answer is E (all). *(Ferrante, p 45.)* Three classes of cells are found in the dorsal horn: (1) projection cells relay information to rostral centers; (2) excitatory interneurons relay nociceptive transmission to projection cells, to other interneurons, or to motor cells concerned with reflexes; and (3) inhibitory interneurons modulate nociceptive transmission. Other cells in the dorsal horn receive additional input from nonnociceptive afferents. These cells are called wide dynamic range (WDR) neurons and respond to a wide range of stimuli from low to high intensity.

80. The answer is C (2,4). *(Ferrante, p 47.)* Laminae I, II, and V are the major areas for convergence of nociceptive transmission at the spinal cord. Cells from these areas project to the thalamus, and cutting this projection abolishes cutaneous pain. Stimulating the projections of laminae I and II produces pain. Discharge of these cells increases with increasing noxious stimulation. In response to a brief noxious stimulus, laminae I and V neurons have early and late discharges, analogous to first and second pain.

81. The answer is E (all). *(Ferrante, p 48.)* The major ascending nociceptive tract in the anterolateral quadrant (ALQ) is the spinothalamic tract (STT). Other tracts of the ALQ that are thought to be involved in pain perception are (1) the spinoreticular tract (SRT), (2) the spinomesencephalic tract (SMT), (3) the dorsal column postsynaptic spinomedullary system, and (4) the propriospinal multisynaptic ascending system.

82. **The answer is E (all).** *(Ferrante, p 51.)* The reticular formation consists of a number of vaguely defined nuclei situated in the core of the brainstem and extending throughout its rostrocaudal aspect. The reticular formation participates in the regulation of motor, sensory, and autonomic functions. Many reticular neurons respond to noxious stimulation, and many respond exclusively to specific noxious modalities. The reticular formation is thought to participate in the affective/motivational component of pain and in the integration of pain with autonomic and motor behavior.

83. **The answer is B (1,3).** *(Ferrante, p 58.)* Evidence implicates serotonin as a neurotransmitter in descending antinociceptive pathways. The rostroventral medulla is rich in serotonergic neurons that project to the spinal cord. Stimulation of neurons in the rostroventral medulla with serotonergic terminals in the dorsal horn inhibits nociceptive neurons in laminae I and II. Application of serotonin to the spinal cord inhibits discharge of spinothalamic tract neurons and relieves pain.

84. **The answer is A (1,2,3).** *(Ferrante, pp 58–59.)* Exogenously administered opioids exert their analgesic effects by acting directly on the CNS. The major anatomic areas involved in opioid-mediated analgesia include the periventricular and periaqueductal gray mattter and the rostroventral medulla.

85. **The answer is C (2,4).** *(Ferrante, p 72.)* The parasympathetic nervous system consists of cranial and sacral portions. The cell bodies of preganglionic parasympathetic fibers are located in cranial nerve nuclei of the brainstem. The long preganglionic fibers of the oculomotor, facial, and glossopharyngeal nerves synapse with short postganglionic fibers of the ciliary, sphenopalatine, and otic ganglia. The very long preganglionic fibers of the vagus synapse in intramural ganglia of the heart, lungs, and gastrointestinal tract. Preganglionic neurons of the sacral portion of the parasympathetic nervous system have cell bodies located in the intermediolateral gray of the second, third, and fourth sacral cord segments.

86. **The answer is A (1,2,3).** *(Ferrante, p 74.)* Acetylcholine is released at all preganglionic nerve endings (both sympathetic and parasympathetic) and postganglionic parasympathetic nerve endings. Sympathetic postganglionic innervation to sweat glands is also cholinergic. Norepinephrine is the neurotransmitter found in postganglionic sympathetic nerve endings.

87. **The answer is C (2,4).** *(Ferrante, p 74.)* Muscarinic receptors are located in all effector cells stimulated by postganglionic parasympathetic neurons as well as postganglionic cholinergic sympathetic neurons. Nicotinic receptors are located in the ganglionic synapses between pre- and postganglionic neurons of the sympathetic and parasympathetic nervous system.

88. **The answer is D (4).** *(Ferrante, p 76.)* The alpha-2 receptors are found in both presynaptic and postsynaptic locations. Stimulation of presynaptic alpha-2 receptors inhibits norepinephrine release, serving as a negative feedback mechanism. Activation of alpha receptors results in increased peripheral vascular resistance, mydriasis, and contraction of pilomotor muscles. Activation of beta receptors results in relaxation of bronchial muscles and increases in cardiac rate and force of contraction.

89. **The answer is E (all).** *(Ferrante, p 147.)* Enkephalins are found in the gastrointestinal tract, sympathetic nervous system, and adrenal medulla. They are found in high density in areas of the CNS important for antinociception: the periaqueductal gray matter, the rostroventral medulla, and Rexed's laminae I, II, V, and X.

90. **The answer is E (all).** *(Ferrante, p 147.)* Beta-endorphin is derived from proopiomelanocortin and is released with adrenocorticotropic hormone (ACTH) from the pituitary. It is the most potent of the endogenous opioids and is found in the hypothalamus, periaqueductal gray matter, and locus ceruleus.

91. **The answer is B (1,3).** *(Ferrante, pp 152–153.)* Activation of kappa receptors causes spinal analgesia but also sedation. Dynorphin is the prototypic endogenous agonist, while ketocyclazocine is the prototypic exogenous agonist. DADL (D-ala, D-leu) is a delta-ligand enkephalin reportedly up to five times more potent than morphine when given in the subarachnoid space, while *N*-allyl normetazocine is a sigma-ligand agonist.

92. **The answer is B (1,3).** *(Ferrante, p 165.)* With continued use of substantial amounts of opioid, the potency of the opioid declines, so that progressively more and more drug is required to produce the same degree of analgesia. This phenomenon, called *tolerance*, is characteristic of opioids as a class of drugs. Tolerance can occur without physical dependence.

93. **The answer is A (1,2,3).** *(Wall, p 247.)* Over 20 different opioid peptides have been identified by biochemical techniques. These peptides are derived from three types of larger prohormones—proopiomelanocortin, proenkephalin A, and proenkephalin B—which are biologically inactive precursors. These large protein molecules are cleaved by proteolytic enzymes within the peptide neuron to form mixtures of smaller peptides. The dynorphins, including alpha-neoendorphin, are formed from proenkephalin B and are intermediate in size.

94. **The answer is C (2,4).** *(Raj, p 592.)* Alpha 1-acid glycoprotein (AAG) has a high affinity for basic drugs but has a low capacity. Albumin has a low affinity but has a high capacity. Because AAG is an acute-phase reactant protein, its abundance in plasma depends on the state of health, recent trauma, and concurrent drug therapy. For example, increases in the plasma concentration of alpha 1-acid glycoprotein occur in response to surgery, chronic pain, rheumatoid arthritis, and acute myocardial infarction.

95. **The answer is B (1,3).** *(Stoelting, p 599.)* Action potentials are conducted from node to node by myelinated nerves rather than continuously along the entire fiber as occurs in the unmyelinated nerve. The successive excitation of nodes of Ranvier by an impulse that jumps between successive nodes is termed *saltatory conduction*. Saltatory conduction greatly increases the velocity of nerve transmission in myelinated fibers and also conserves energy because only the nodes of Ranvier depolarize, resulting in lower loss of ions than would otherwise occur.

96. **The answer is A (1,2,3).** *(Stoelting, p 599.)* The neuron consists of a cell body (soma), dendrites, and an axon (nerve fiber). Dendrites are extensions of the cell body. The axon of one neuron terminates near the cell body or dendrites of another neuron. A synapse is the junction between neurons and serves as an important control mechanism for transmission of impulses.

97. **The answer is E (all).** *(Stoelting, p 601.)* The five basic types of sensory receptors are (1) nociceptors, which detect painful stimuli due to physical or chemical damage in tissue; (2) mechanoreceptors, which detect tissue deformation; (3) thermoreceptors for cold and warmth; (4) electromagnetic receptors, which detect light on the retina; and (5) chemoreceptors, which detect taste, smell, arterial partial pressure of oxygen and carbon dioxide, and serum osmolarity.

98. **The answer is B (1,3).** *(Stoelting, p 601.)* Glycine is secreted mainly at synapses in the spinal cord, where it functions predominantly as an inhibitory neurotransmitter. GABA is an inhibitory neurotransmitter secreted by neurons in diverse areas of the nervous system including the spinal cord, cerebellum, and basal ganglia. Glutamic acid is an excitatory neurotransmitter secreted by many of the sensory pathways of the CNS. Substance P is also an excitatory neurotransmitter presumed to be released by terminals of pain fibers in the substantia gelatinosa of the spinal cord.

99. **The answer is B (1,3).** *(Stoelting, p 604.)* Neurons are highly responsive to changes in the pH of the surrounding interstitial fluids. Alkalosis enhances neuronal excitability as does hyperventilation. Acidosis depresses neuron excitability. Lack of oxygen can cause total inexcitability of neurons within 3 to 5 s.

100. **The answer is D (4).** *(Stoelting, p 607.)* Withdrawal flexor reflexes are most often elicited by a painful stimulus. Pathways for eliciting the withdrawal reflex do not pass directly to the anterior motor neurons but instead pass first through several interneurons. Associated with withdrawal of the stimulated limb is extension of the opposite limb, which occurs 0.2 to 0.5 s later and serves to push the body away from the object causing the painful stimulus.

101. The answer is C (2,4). *(Tollison, p 239.)* Pain-sensitive structures include such intracranial structures as the cranial sinuses and afferent veins, the arteries of the dura mater, the arteries of the base of the brain and their major branches, and parts of the dura mater in the vicinity of large vessels. Extracranial structures that are pain-sensitive include the skin, scalp, fascia, muscles, mucosa, arteries, and veins. The trigeminal, facial, vagal, glossopharyngeal, and second and third cranial nerves are also sensitive.

Structures insensitive to pain include the intracranial structures of the parenchyma of the brain, ependyma, choroid plexus, pia mater, arachnoid membrane, and parts of the dura mater, as well as the extracranial skull (except for the periosteum, which is slightly pain-sensitive).

102. The answer is A (1,2,3). *(Ferrante, pp 152–153.)* Activation of mu-1 receptors has analgesic effects (mostly supraspinal, though some mu-1 receptors are found in the spinal cord). Activation of mu-2 receptors produces respiratory depression, bradycardia, and depression of GI motility. Spinal analgesia is mediated by the delta and kappa receptors. Kappa-receptor activation results in spinal analgesia and sedation without respiratory depression. Delta-receptor activation results in spinal analgesia without sedation or respiratory depression. The delta-receptor ligand (D-ala, D-leu enkephalin; DADL) has been found to be five times more potent than morphine (a mu-receptor agonist) when given intrathecally. Sigma-receptor stimulation produces dysphoria, hallucinations, tachycardia, tachypnea, and mydriasis.

103. The answer is E (all). *(Wall, pp 211–212, 227.)* All peripheral nerve injury appears to have a central effect. After peripheral nerve injury, the primary afferents arborize into new areas of the dorsal horn. In addition, they stop making substance P and CGRP and start making neuropeptide y, galanin, and VIP. There is upregulation of the early immediate gene C-Fos, which stimulates production of Fos protein and increased production of dynorphin by second-order neurons.

104. The answer is C (2,4). *(Ferrante, pp 147–150.)* Endogenous opioids modulate nociception. All endogenous opioids contain the amino acid sequence tyrosine-glycine-phenylalanine. They are cleaved from three precursor molecules: proenkephalin A, proopiomelanocortin, and prodynorphin (proenkephalin B). Proenkephalin A is cleaved to form met- and leu-enkephalins. Enkephalins are found in highest concentration in the GI tract, sympathetic nervous system, adrenal medulla, periaqueductal gray, the rostroventral medulla, and Rexed's laminae I, II, V, and X. Beta-endorphin, which is derived from proopiomelanocortin, is released from the pituitary gland along with ACTH. It is the most potent opioid and is found in high concentrations in the hypothalamus, periaqueductal gray, and locus ceruleus. Prodynorphin is cleaved to form dynorphin and alpha-neoendorphin, which are not potent analgesics. They are found in the same distribution as the enkephalins. Their function has not been fully determined.

105. The answer is C (2,4). *(Ramamurthy, p 20.)* A-delta fibers are myelinated fibers that transmit sharp pain, temperature, and possibly touch. C fibers are unmyelinated fibers that transmit the sensation of dull pain, temperature, and touch. A-beta fibers carry small motor, touch, and pressure sensation. B fibers are preganglionic autonomic fibers.

106. The answer is A (1,2,3). *(Cousins, p 271.)* The large, valveless epidural veins are part of the internal vertebral venous plexus, which drains the neural tissue of the spinal cord, CSF, and the bony spiny canal. The major portion of this plexus lies in the anterolateral part of the epidural space, out of reach of a correctly placed epidural needle. By way of the intervertebral foramina at each level, the vertebral plexus communicates with thoracic and abdominal veins. Thus, marked increases in intraabdominal pressure may compress the inferior vena cava while distending the epidural veins and increasing flow up the vertebrobasilar plexus.

107. The answer is A (1,2,3). *(Cousins, p 551.)* The deep cervical plexus is composed of the C2–C4 spinal nerves as they emerge from the foramina in the cervical vertebrae. Traditionally blockade is performed using a three-needle technique. Insertion sites are located by reference to a line that joins the tip of the mastoid process with Chassaignac's tubercle of C6, which is palpated at the level of the cricoid cartilage. The posterior border of the sternocleidomastoid muscle is the major point of reference used in performing blockade of the superficial cervical plexus.

108. **The answer is C (2,4).** *(Cousins, pp 581–582.)* Six extraocular muscles control the movements of the eye. The four rectus muscles (superior, medial, inferior, and lateral) originate from a common tendon ring that encircles the optic foramen. The superior oblique muscle originates above and medial to the optic foramen, while the inferior oblique muscle originates medially from the periosteum of the lacrimal bone. The oculomotor nerve (CN III) innervates the superior, medial, and inferior rectus muscles as well as the inferior oblique and levator palpebrae superioris muscles. The lateral rectus muscle is innervated by the abducens nerve (CN VI) while the superior oblique muscle receives innervation from the trochlear nerve (CN IV).

109. **The answer is C (2,4).** *(Bonica, p 961.)* The first seven pairs of the 12 ribs are known as the *vertebrosternal ribs*. They connect dorsally with the vertebral column and ventrally with the sternum by means of costal cartilages. The remaining five pairs are "false" ribs and consist of two types. The 8th to 10th ribs have their cartilages attached to the cartilage of the rib above (vertebrochondral), while the 11th and 12th ribs are free at their anterior extremities and are referred to as *floating* or *vertebral ribs* because they do not attach to the sternum.

110. **The answer is A (1,2,3).** *(Bonica, p 962.)* The ligamenta flava connect the laminae of adjacent vertebrae. Each ligamentum flavum consists of yellow elastic tissue attached to the anterior and inferior surfaces of the lamina above and to the posterior superior surface of the lamina below. The fibers of the ligamenta flava are oriented perpendicularly to the laminae to which they are attached. They are thin in the cervical region, thicker in the thoracic region, and thickest in the lumbar region.

111. **The answer is C (2,4).** *(Bonica, p 965.)* The most central portion of the diaphragm is innervated by the phrenic nerves, which arise from the two cervical plexuses (C3–C5), while the diaphragm's peripheral muscular fibers are supplied by the 6th to the 11th or 12th intercostal nerves.

112. **The answer is B (1,3).** *(Bonica, p 967.)* The intercostal nerves are distributed chiefly to the thorax and abdomen. They differ from other spinal nerves in that each pursues an independent course and, except for the first intercostal nerve, they do not enter into the formation of plexuses. The smaller posterior primary divisions diverge from their anterior counterparts and run posteriorly to supply the muscles and skin of the back through medial and lateral branches.

113. **The answer is C (2,4).** *(Bonica, p 982.)* The visceral pleura is supplied by sympathetic fibers that have a vasomotor function. It has afferent fibers that do not have a nociceptive function, making it insensitive to noxious stimuli. It also receives parasympathetic fibers through the pulmonary plexuses. The parietal pleura is supplied by the intercostal nerves at its lateral aspects, by the T1 spinal nerve at its apex, and by the phrenic nerves on the diaphragmatic surface.

114. **The answer is A (1,2,3).** *(Bonica, p 1150.)* The abdominal wall is divided into nine regions by four imaginary lines of which two pass horizontally around the body and two vertically. The upper horizontal line (transpyloric plane) lies between the suprasternal notch and the symphysis pubis. The lower line (transtubercular plane) lies at the top of the crests of the iliac bones. Two vertical lines (one on each side of the body) descend from the cartilages of the 8th rib to the center of the inguinal ligament. The nine regions include the right and left hypochondriac, lumbar, and iliac areas and in the midline the epigastric, umbilical, and hypogastric areas.

115. **The answer is E (all).** *(Bonica, p 1156.)* The celiac plexus is composed of two or more large aggregates of ganglion cells, the right and left celiac ganglia, a number of smaller ganglia, and a dense network of parasympathetic and sympathetic efferent and afferent fibers that enmesh these ganglia. The plexus is situated in the epigastrium just anterior to the crura of the diaphragm and the body of the first lumbar vertebra. The entire plexus lies posterior to the stomach and the omental bursa.

116. **The answer is A (1,2,3).** *(Bonica, p 1298.)* The somatic fibers of the pudendal nerve are derived from the anterior primary divisions of the S2, S3, and S4 nerves, while the sympathetic fibers are contributed by the sacral portion of the sympathetic chain. The formed nerve leaves the pelvic cavity by passing through the greater sciatic foramen inferior to the piriformis muscle, between it and the coccygeal muscle. The pudendal nerve trunk divides into three main branches: the inferior hemorrhoidal nerve, the perineal nerve, and the dorsal nerve to the clitoris (or to the penis).

117. **The answer is C (2,4).** *(Bonica, p 1397.)* The posterior longitudinal ligament (PLL) extends along the posterior surface of the body of the vertebra from the cervical axis to the sacrum and contributes to the anterior wall of the vertebral canal. The PLL is broad throughout the length of the vertebral column until it reaches the L1 vertebral level, where it begins to narrow progressively so that at the L5–S1 interspace it is only half its original width. The PLL is composed of longitudinal fibers that are denser and more compact than those of the anterior longitudinal ligament.

118. **The answer is A (1,2,3).** *(Bonica, p 1400.)* Early in life, the blood supply to the disk is from the periphery as well as from vessels in the bodies of adjacent vertebrae, which grow through the cartilaginous plates and run toward but do not reach the nucleus pulposus. Shortly after birth, the vascular supply begins to diminish and by the third decade of life, the disk is almost avascular. Thereafter, it receives nutrients by diffusion of solutes, lymph, and other fluids through the cervical portion, the vertebral end plate, and the annulus fibrosus. This is made possible by alternating compression and relaxation of the elastic container.

119. **The answer is C (2,4).** *(Bonica, p 1400.)* The posterior articulations (or facets) comprise two arthrodial joints lined with synovium and lubricated with synovial fluid. The orientation of the facets determines the direction of motion of that spinal segment. In the thoracic spine, the facets are convex-concave and lie in the horizontal plane, permitting lateral flexing, side bending, and rotation about a vertical line. In the upper lumbar spine, the facets lie in a vertical sagittal plane and permit flexion and extension but prevent lateral flexion or bending in the lordotic curve.

120. **The answer is E (all).** *(Bonica, p 1411.)* The epidural space is bound anteriorly by the posterior longitudinal ligament and the vertebral bodies, and laterally by the pedicles and intervertebral foramina. Posterior boundaries of the epidural space include the laminae and ligamenta flava, while its inferior boundary is its continuation with the sacral canal. The size of the epidural space varies greatly. The anterior portion is the narrowest (approximately 1 mm). In the lumbar region, the epidural space is triangular with the apex of the triangle corresponding to the posterior midline of the vertebral canal.

121. **The answer is B (1,3).** *(Bonica, p 264.)* Neural (neurogenic) pain differs from nociceptive pain in several ways. Typically, its onset is delayed after a causative event and it is often causalgic or dysesthetic in nature. Neurogenic pain may respond to intravenous administration of barbiturate-like drugs but usually not to opiates. It is usually temporarily relieved by proximal local anesthetic blockade but not permanently relieved by surgical interruption at the same site.

122. **The answer is A (1,2,3).** *(Raj, p 83.)* Exteroceptive sensations are those that arise from or originate in sense organs in the skin or mucous membranes and respond to external agents and changes in the environment. They may also be designated as *superficial sensations*. There are three major types: pain, temperature, and touch.

123. **The answer is B (1,3).** *(Raj, p 89.)* To elicit the corneal reflex, the examiner touches the cornea lightly with a wisp of cotton, a piece of string, or a hair. In response to this stimulus, there is a blinking or closing of the ipsilateral eye (i.e., the direct corneal reflex) as well as a closing of the opposite eye (i.e., the consensual corneal reflex). The afferent limb of the reflex is the ophthalmic division of the trigeminal nerve (CN V); the efferent limb is mediated by the facial nerve (CN VII), which conveys the impulse to the orbicularis oculi.

124. **The answer is A (1,2,3).** *(Raj, p 108.)* Stroking the skin on the upper, inner aspect of the thigh elicits the cremaster reflex. The response consists of a contraction of the cremasteric muscle, with ipsilateral elevation of the testicle. The innervation is through the L1 and L2 segments (ilioinguinal and genitofemoral nerves).

Diagnostic Testing

DIRECTIONS: Each question below contains suggested responses. Select the **one best** response.

125. The F wave is correctly described by which of the following statements?

    (A) It is a true reflex
    (B) It occurs before the M wave
    (C) It can only be measured in the lower extremity
    (D) It requires adequate spinal cord and peripheral nerve function

126. All the following statements are true regarding the H wave that is obtained during electrodiagnostic evaluation EXCEPT that

    (A) it is the electrical equivalent of the deep tendon reflex of the ankle
    (B) it is a polysynaptic reflex response
    (C) the latency of the response is affected by age
    (D) an abnormal H wave indicates neural dysfunction in the spinal cord, spinal nerve root, or tibial nerve

127. A complete electrodiagnostic evaluation would include all the following EXCEPT

    (A) electromyography and late response studies
    (B) peripheral nerve conduction studies of motor and sensory nerves
    (C) muscle biopsy
    (D) somatosensory evoked potentials

128. The diagnosis of carpal tunnel syndrome would be supported by all the following electrodiagnostic studies EXCEPT

    (A) normal needle EMG
    (B) abnormal ulnar nerve conduction velocities
    (C) normal ulnar F-wave conduction
    (D) Prolonged median nerve sensory latency

129. A 26-year-old construction worker injured his back while picking up lumber 6 months prior to evaluation at the pain clinic. Bed rest, NSAIDs, and muscle relaxants did not provide significant relief. The patient now complains of chronic pain and weakness of his right leg. On physical examination, atrophy of the thigh and calf muscles is noted, as well as an absent deep tendon reflex of the right ankle and 2/5 motor strength. There is diminished sensation most pronounced at the lateral aspect of his foot.

    Electrodiagnostic studies were ordered. Which of the following findings would be consistent with his physical examination?

    (A) Normal needle EMG of the medial gastrocnemius
    (B) Normal needle EMG of the lateral hamstrings
    (C) Normal H-wave latency
    (D) Normal needle EMG of the adductor longus

Questions 130–131

130. A 36-year-old woman with pelvic pain of unknown etiology (despite extensive evaluation) underwent a differential epidural block. After no response to 5 mL of 0.9% saline, a total of 10 mL of 0.5% lidocaine was administered. Her sensation to pain was intact, with a 2°C rise in skin temperature and a marked decrease in her pain. This response suggests

(A) placebo response
(B) sympathetic-mediated pain
(C) somatic cause of pain
(D) psychogenic pain

131. Another block that could be performed to confirm the results of the differential epidural block would be

(A) splanchnic block
(B) lumbar sympathetic block
(C) hypogastric plexus block
(D) celiac plexus block

---

132. During an intravenous lidocaine test, all the following monitors are recommended EXCEPT

(A) electrocardiography
(B) skin temperature
(C) blood pressure
(D) pulse oximetry

133. Thermography can be used for all the following purposes EXCEPT to

(A) document the locations of myofascial trigger points
(B) evaluate sympathetic blockade after stellate ganglion block
(C) prove the presence of psychogenic pain syndromes
(D) support the diagnosis of reflex sympathetic dystrophy

134. A 46-year-old factory worker complains of disabling low back pain. Physical examination and testing failed to reveal any abnormalities. A thiopental (Pentothal) test was performed. Straight leg raising to 60° caused pain while the patient was awake and caused grimacing with withdrawal movements during the thiopental test. This response suggests that

(A) there is likely to be peripheral pathology
(B) surgery is unlikely to benefit the patient
(C) the patient is malingering
(D) psychotherapy may be helpful

135. To evaluate warm temperature sensation, the stimulus should be in which of the following temperature ranges?

(A) 25 to 29°C (77 to 84.2°F)
(B) 30 to 35°C (86 to 95°F)
(C) 36 to 39°C (96.8 to 102.2°F)
(D) 40 to 45°C (104 to 113°F)

136. In the examination of temperature sensation, a cold stimulus ideally should be

(A) −5 to 0°C (23 to 32°F)
(B) 0 to 5°C (32 to 41°F)
(C) 5 to 10°C (41 to 50°F)
(D) 10 to 15°C (50 to 59°F)
(E) 15 to 20°C (59 to 68°F)

137. You suspect arterial insufficiency in a patient complaining of a painful lower extremity. His ankle brachial index is 0.4. What would be the most appropriate treatment for this patient?

(A) Rest, elevation of the limb, and NSAIDs
(B) Medication to control high blood pressure or hyperglycemia, regular exercise, and cessation of smoking
(C) Referral to a vascular specialist
(D) Vasodilator medications and narcotic analgesics
(E) Epidural steroids and physical therapy

138. Which of the following statements is true?

    (A) Electromyographic changes occur within 24 h of neural injury
    (B) Testing of neural conduction velocity is more sensitive than electromyography in the early stages of neural injury
    (C) Increased motor potential in muscle groups occurs with neural injury
    (D) Increased neural conduction velocity occurs with neural injury
    (E) Changes in neural conduction velocity take weeks to become apparent after neural injury

139. Magnetic resonance imaging (MRI) is superior to computed tomography (CT) in the diagnosis of which type of intracranial lesion?

    (A) Parental lobe abscess
    (B) Frontal lobe neoplasms
    (C) Cerebral edema
    (D) Cerebral hemorrhage
    (E) Lesions of the posterior fossa and brainstem

140. Which of the following has been found to be a perpetuator of myofascial trigger points in many patients?

    (A) Low vitamin B_{12} or folate
    (B) High bilirubin
    (C) Low serum creatinine
    (D) Low cholesterol
    (E) Low vitamin D

DIRECTIONS: Each question below contains four suggested responses of which **one or more** is correct. Select

A	if	**1, 2, and 3**	are correct
B	if	**1 and 3**	are correct
C	if	**2 and 4**	are correct
D	if	**4**	is correct
E	if	**1, 2, 3, and 4**	are correct

141. Which of the following may be responsible for a false positive response after a diagnostic regional block?

    (1) Systemic effects of local anesthetic
    (2) Unreliable patient's report of the effects of the block
    (3) Placebo response
    (4) Effects of peripheral block on central processing

142. What positive information can be derived from an epidural diagnostic nerve block?

    (1) Sympathetic versus somatic pain can be determined
    (2) The segmental level of nociceptive input may be established
    (3) Psychogenic versus somatic pain can be determined
    (4) Continuation of pain below an area fully blocked suggests pain of a higher central focus

143. A patient has more than 50 percent relief of pain after infusion of intravenous lidocaine. This response suggests that it would be reasonable to place the patient on which of the following medications?

    (1) Tocainide
    (2) Phenytoin
    (3) Mexiletine
    (4) Methadone

144. Which of the following can be used to perform the sweating test, a special test of the function of the autonomic nervous system?

    (1) Cobalt blue papers
    (2) Iodine in oil and starch powder
    (3) Ferric chloride and tannic acid
    (4) Pilocarpine hydrochloride

145. Which of the following diagnostic studies will provide more information regarding the spinal cord and nerve roots than unenhanced computed tomography (CT)?

    (1) Magnetic resonance imaging (MRI)
    (2) Myelography
    (3) Intrathecally enhanced CT
    (4) Oblique plain films

Diagnostic Testing

Answers

125. **The answer is D.** *(Bonica, p 628.)* The F wave is a late response that occurs after stimulation of motor nerves in the upper and lower extremities. The initial response to stimulation of motor nerves is the M wave; this is followed by the late response F wave when approximately 5 percent of the motor neurons stimulated "rebound." The rebound occurs because some of the anterior horn cell refractory periods are shorter than the duration of the stimulus and thus will "refire" and produce the late response F wave. F waves are not true reflexes like H waves. Because the rebound occurs at spinal cord level, in order to obtain a normal F wave, both spinal cord and peripheral nerve function must be intact.

126. **The answer is B.** *(Bonica, p 627.)* H-wave responses are late responses that occur after peripheral stimulation has produced an action potential and has traveled to the spinal cord or brainstem and returned to the stimulation site. H-wave responses, in adults, are only obtainable in the lower extremities. H waves are true reflexes (F waves are not.) The H-wave response is a monosynaptic reflex that occurs when the tibial nerve is stimulated and is the electrical equivalent of the deep tendon reflex of the ankle. The tibial nerve is stimulated behind the knee and impulses travel via 1A afferent fibers to the spinal cord at the S1 level. After synapse in the cord, the anterior horn cells produce a motor response, which can be recorded by surface electrodes in the gastrocnemius and soleus muscles. Response latency is affected by age. Disease or trauma to the tibial nerve, S1 nerve root, or spinal cord will produce an abnormal H wave.

127. **The answer is C.** *(Bonica, p 629.)* The electromyogram (EMG), peripheral nerve conduction studies (NCSs), late response studies, and somatosensory evoked potentials (SEPs) help to characterize the nature and location of the abnormality being studied. Determination of the cause of the abnormality can occur only after integration of the information obtained from the physical examination, history, and electrodiagnostic and radiologic studies. Muscle biopsy is not a component of electrodiagnostic evaluation.

128. **The answer is B.** *(Bonica, pp 631–632.)* A normal needle EMG is possible in patients with carpal tunnel syndrome. It indicates the absence of a motor radiculopathy. Normal ulnar nerve studies should be present. Abnormal studies of the median nerve that are likely to be present in patients with carpal tunnel syndrome and support its diagnosis include prolonged sensory and motor distal latencies, decreased sensory amplitudes, and decreased motor conduction velocity of the median nerve. With prolonged, severe cases, motor nerve axonal degeneration may occur and would result in abnormal needle EMG examination of the muscles supplied by the ulnar nerve.

129. **The answer is D.** *(Bonica, p 634.)* The patient has a clinical picture consistent with an S1 radiculopathy. Abnormal EMG findings would be expected for those muscles with S1 innervation such as the lateral hamstrings, medial and lateral gastrocnemius (S1,L5), anterior tibialis, extensor hallucis longus, tensor fascia

lata, and medial hamstrings (L5,S1), but not for the vastus medialis, rectus femoris, and adductor longus, which are innervated by L4,L3. The H-wave late response is a useful test for S1 involvement and would be prolonged or have a markedly decreased amplitude in patients with S1 radiculopathy.

130. **The answer is B.** *(Ramamurthy, p 20.)* Differential epidural or spinal blockade is possible because of the differential sensitivity of the nerve fibers to local anesthetics. The most sensitive fibers are the B fibers (preganglionic autonomic fibers). The next most sensitive are the A-delta and C fibers, which are responsible for sharp and dull pain and touch. The least sensitive are the larger A fibers, which supply muscle tone and motor function. In this case, the patient responded to a very dilute anesthetic, with preservation of touch and signs of autonomic blockade. This response supports the diagnosis of a pain syndrome with a sympathetic-mediated component.

131. **The answer is C.** *(Raj, pp 813–817.)* Hypogastric plexus blockade is useful in blocking pelvic pain due to autonomic dysfunction. The hypogastric plexus is formed by postganglionic sympathetic fibers, preganglionic parasympathetic fibers, and visceral afferent fibers. It is located at the anterior aspect of the 5th lumbar vertebra, just inferior to the aortic bifurcation.

132. **The answer is B.** *(Ramamurthy, pp 18–19.)* Intravenous lidocaine can be used to determine the efficacy of treatment with oral antiarrhythmics such as mexiletine or tocainide. It may be used as a treatment itself if weekly infusions provide longer relief after each treatment. Some studies suggest that intravenous lidocaine may have predictive value as to the efficacy of anticonvulsants such as phenytoin or carbamazepine. Because of the possibility of systemic toxicity and seizures, patients should be monitored by electrocardiography, blood pressure, and pulse oximetry. Skin temperature monitoring is not necessary. Resuscitation equipment must be available.

133. **The answer is C.** *(Ramamurthy, p 14.)* In clinical practice, thermography is useful only as a means to measure skin temperature over a wide body area. It has been used to diagnose reflex sympathetic dystrophy, entrapment neuropathies, spinal nerve root irritation, vascular disease, joint disease, and fractures. It has also been used to evaluate the degree of sympathetic blockade after stellate ganglion, lumbar sympathetic, or epidural blocks. Thermography can also document locations of myofascial trigger points.

134. **The answer is A.** *(Ramamurthy, pp 16–17.)* Thiopental (Pentothal) testing may be useful in the evaluation of patients who present a diagnostic dilemma. Patients who complain of pain out of proportion to clinical findings may have significant psychological overlay. In some instances, the thiopental test may help to clarify whether there is an organic cause of the patient's pain. The patient is given thiopental sodium in 50-mg increments per minute until loss of the lash reflex and loss of voice response. Movements that had previously caused the patient to complain of pain are repeated. Physical response, such as grimacing or withdrawal behaviors, suggests peripheral pathology, which warrants further investigation and possible surgical or conventional medical therapies. Lack of physical response suggests that the patient may have central or psychogenic pain or may be malingering.

135. **The answer is D.** *(Raj, p 84.)* To test warm temperature sensation, a glass or metal tube containing hot water with a temperature in the range of 40 to 45°C (104 to 113°F) should be used. Temperatures higher than 45°C are perceived as painful.

136. **The answer is C.** *(Raj, p 84.)* For quantitative evaluation of temperature sensation, a thermophore may be used. For testing cold, the stimulus should be 5 to 10°C (41 to 50°F); for testing warmth, from 40 to 45°C (104 to 113°F). Temperatures much lower or higher than these elicit the sensation of pain rather than of temperature.

137. The answer is C. *(Bonica, pp 503–505.)* A simple noninvasive pressure measurement to evaluate a patient with suspected arterial insufficiency can be obtained by determining the ankle systolic pressure with a Doppler ultrasound instrument and comparing it to brachial systolic pressure. Normal ankle systolic pressure is equal to or greater than the brachial systolic pressure (ankle brachial index, ABI ≥ 1.0). If arterial insufficiency is present, the ABI will be less than 1.0. Patients with mild insufficiency have an ABI between 0.5 and 0.7; those with severe disease have an ABI less than 0.5. An ABI of 0.4 will most likely require surgical evaluation and treatment. Ischemic ulcers will not heal and gangrene may occur.

Other noninvasive vascular studies include plethysmography, Doppler flow velocity tracings, skin temperature measurements, and thermography. A semi-invasive diagnostic test for peripheral vascular disease is injection of isotope intravascularly or into tissue to assess radioactive clearance and distribution. Invasive tests can also be performed, such as the intraarterial placement of an electromagnetic flow meter or ultrasonic velocity detector. Angiography, arteriography, venography, and lymphography are usually performed only if surgery is being considered.

138. The answer is B. *(Tollison, p 326.)* If neural injury is suspected, electromyography and testing of neural conduction velocity can provide information as to the extent and location of injury. With neural injury, a decrease in motor potential in muscle groups and slowed conduction velocities occur. Neural conduction velocities are decreased quickly after neural injury. Electromyographic changes may take weeks to occur. Therefore, testing of neural conduction velocity is more sensitive than electromyography in the early stages of neural injury.

139. The answer is E. *(Tollison, p 242.)* Lesions of the posterior fossa and brainstem are best visualized by MRI. They are difficult to identify on CT because of bone artifact. CT is the method used to identify most incranial lesions, including neoplasms, abscesses, and hematomas. It can detect hydrocephalus, cerebral edema, infarction, hemorrhage, and arteriovenous malformations.

140. The answer is A. *(Tollison, pp 525–526.)* Low serum levels of vitamin B_{12} or folate or both have been found to be associated with increased trigger points in many patients who suffer from myofascial pain syndrome. To rule out underlying systemic diseases that may cause or exacerbate myofascial pain, other laboratory tests should also be performed, such as a complete blood count screen; measurement of erythrocyte sedimentation rate and levels of uric acid, potassium, calcium, cholesterol, vitamin A, B_1, B_6, and ascorbic acid; and thyroid function tests.

141. The answer is E (all). *(Cousins, p 896.)* False positive responses arise when pain reduction is inferred as being a specific consequence of the block when in fact pain reduction is due to some action other than that intended or supposed. Possible explanations for this result include placebo response, an unreliable patient's report of the effect of the block, effects of local anesthetic absorbed into the circulation, and effects of peripheral block on central processing.

142. The answer is C (2,4). *(Cousins, p 893.)* There is no way to be certain of producing a "pure" block of sympathetic, sensory, or motor fibers. When performing a classic "differential" block, spinal or epidural diagnostic local anesthetic blockade may establish the segmental level of nociceptive input. In addition, continuation of pain in or below an area fully blocked suggests pain of a higher central focus.

143. The answer is A (1,2,3). *(Ramamurthy, pp 18–19.)* The analgesic effect of lidocaine is thought to be anesthesia of small nerve endings in regions of tissue injury as well as interruption of C-fiber synaptic transmission in the spinal cord. If patients have a good analgesic response to lidocaine, they may benefit from oral therapy using tocainide or mexiletine. There are also data to suggest that the response to anticonvulsant medications such as phenytoin and carbamazepine can be predicted by the response to intravenous infusion of lidocaine.

144. The answer is E (all). *(Raj, pp 117–120.)* Observation and physical examination of the patient provide substantial information about the function of the autonomic nervous system. Evaluation of endocrine status, body temperature, vital signs, skin and mucous membranes, perspiration, hair and nail growth, salivation, lacrimation, and extremities, as well as documentation of autonomic reflexes involving the cranial nerves should be performed prior to special tests of autonomic function. Several tests exist to supplement the information obtained on examination of the patient. The sweating test will reveal areas of autonomic dysfunction. Cobalt blue papers will turn pink when exposed to moisture and will remain blue in areas of anhidrosis. Iodine in oil will turn bluish black in the presence of starch and moisture. Ferric chloride turns black in the presence of tannic acid and moisture. Sweating can be elicited by application of external heat, ingestion of hot fluids and aspirin, emotional stimuli, intellectual strain, painful cutaneous sensation, or subcutaneous injection of 5 mg of pilocarpine hydrochloride.

Other tests of autonomic function include assessment of the pilomotor response, vasomotor response, reflex erythema, histamine flare, skin temperature, skin resistance, capillary microscopy, and plethysmography.

145. The answer is A (1,2,3). *(Tollison, p 326.)* Plain films are useful to show bony pathology. Flexion and extension views provide information regarding spinal stability. Oblique views allow visualization of the neural foramina. Unenhanced CT provides detailed visualization of bony anatomy. In the past, myelography was the best method to evaluate the spinal cord and nerve roots. However, this method is rapidly being replaced by MRI or intrathecally enhanced CT.

Types of Pain

DIRECTIONS: Each question below contains suggested responses. Select the **one best** response.

146. Pain is best defined as

    (A) the response to a stimulus that is damaging to tissue integrity
    (B) the process of detecting and signaling the presence of a noxious stimulus
    (C) the emotional reaction of an organism to a noxious stimulus
    (D) an unpleasant sensory and emotional experience associated with actual or potential tissue damage or described in terms of such damage

147. Diminished biceps and brachioradialis reflexes associated with numbness and weakness of the deltoid are due to compression of which nerve root?

    (A) C5
    (B) C6
    (C) C7
    (D) C8

148. A 26-year-old weight lifter felt a sharp pain in the neck, radiating to the dorsal aspect of the forearm during his workout. Over the next few days he noted progressive numbness of the thumb and index finger. He also complained of decreased ability to perform bicep curls. On examination by his primary care doctor, a markedly diminished biceps reflex was found. Which of the following is the most likely cause of the patient's problem?

    (A) Fractured C5 vertebra
    (B) C5–C6 disk protrusion
    (C) Facet syndrome at C5–C6
    (D) Compression of the C5 nerve root by an osteophyte

149. Allodynia can be defined as

    (A) hypersensitivity to a painful stimulus
    (B) summation of mildly painful stimuli that causes severe pain
    (C) pain caused by a nonpainful stimulus
    (D) pain present in an area of numbness

150. Which of the following is typically the most difficult type of pain to treat?

    (A) Psychogenic pain
    (B) Intermittent somatic pain
    (C) Continuous visceral pain
    (D) Intermittent neuropathic pain
    (E) Chronic pain

151. All the following are examples of nociceptive types of pain EXCEPT

    (A) inflammation
    (B) distended viscera
    (C) fractures
    (D) phantom limb pain
    (E) lacerations

152. All the following are true regarding nociceptive pain EXCEPT

    (A) it is not commonly relieved by narcotic agents
    (B) it is described as sharp or shooting in nature
    (C) it may be relieved by changing position
    (D) it is described as intermittent, cramping, and throbbing
    (E) it is commonly abolished by local anesthetic blockade

153. A 35-year-old construction worker presents with a chief complaint of pain over the dorsal aspect of the forearm and inability to fully extend the arm at the elbow. Physical examination reveals diminished sensation over the dorsal aspect of the index and middle fingers as well as an absent triceps reflex. Which of the following nerve roots is most likely involved?

    (A) C5
    (B) C6
    (C) C7
    (D) C8
    (E) T1

154. All the following are true regarding visceral pain EXCEPT

    (A) traction and distention usually produce pain
    (B) cutting and burning usually produce pain
    (C) pain can commonly be referred
    (D) pain is diffuse and poorly localized
    (E) viscera have fewer nociceptors than somatic structures

155. Ramsay Hunt syndrome (herpes zoster oticus) occurs when herpes zoster involves the

    (A) gasserian ganglion
    (B) sphenopalatine ganglion
    (C) ciliary ganglion
    (D) geniculate ganglion
    (E) trigeminal nerve

156. Temporal arteritis is correctly described by all the following EXCEPT

    (A) a swollen, tender scalp artery is present
    (B) it is frequently accompanied by polymyalgia rheumatica
    (C) patients usually have an elevated erythrocyte sedimentation rate (ESR)
    (D) there are typical histologic features on biopsy
    (E) it is not responsive to steroid therapy

157. All the following statements regarding endometriosis are correct EXCEPT that the pain

    (A) is characteristically worse during menstruation
    (B) may mimic acute appendicitis
    (C) may result from a direct action on nerve endings
    (D) may be resolved with NSAIDs
    (E) is commonly felt in the hypogastric region

158. The uncommon Sluder's neuralgia, characterized by severe pain in the face below the eyebrows, primarily involves the

    (A) gasserian ganglion
    (B) sphenopalatine ganglion
    (C) ciliary ganglion
    (D) geniculate ganglion
    (E) trigeminal nerve

159. Which of the following types of headaches is most likely to be responsive to inhalation of 100% oxygen?

    (A) Migraine headache
    (B) Tension headache
    (C) Cluster headache
    (D) Cervicogenic headache
    (E) Chronic paroxysmal hemicrania

160. All the following statements regarding a spinal epidural abscess are true EXCEPT that

    (A) the most common symptom is back pain
    (B) symptoms may not occur for 1 to 2 weeks following a medical procedure
    (C) it commonly leads to radicular symptoms
    (D) paraplegia can result
    (E) it most commonly results from inadequate cleaning of the skin

161. All the following are true regarding tension headaches EXCEPT that they

    (A) occur mostly in men
    (B) are commonly associated with sleep disturbance
    (C) often occur bilaterally
    (D) do not have a hereditary pattern
    (E) evolve over hours to days

162. Which of the following is the LEAST likely location to develop an acute herpes zoster infection?

    (A) Face
    (B) Lumbar dermatome
    (C) Sacral dermatome
    (D) Thoracic dermatome
    (E) Cervical dermatome

163. A patient complains of S1 radicular pain on straight-leg raising to 30°. Crossed straight-leg raising caused the same pain. These findings on physical examination support a diagnosis of

    (A) L5–S1 disk herniation
    (B) facet arthropathy
    (C) sciatica
    (D) malingering

164. A previously healthy 27-year-old woman presents to the emergency ward with a complaint of generalized muscular pain with aching in the left buttock for 1 week. The pain travels down the back of her leg to the heel and lateral side of her foot to the small toe. She has also noted a progressive numbness in her legs and arms, which has worsened over the week. She came in to the emergency ward for new onset of leg weakness. Walking is very difficult, and her legs buckle when she stands. The most likely diagnosis is

    (A) postherpetic neuralgia
    (B) brain tumor
    (C) hysterical reaction
    (D) Guillain-Barré syndrome

165. Which of the following statements regarding the pain of multiple sclerosis (MS) is true?

    (A) Trigeminal neuralgia is the most common pain disorder associated with MS
    (B) Most patients with MS have headaches associated with the disease process
    (C) Primary psychogenic pain is common in MS
    (D) The majority of MS patients with pain have central pain associated with the disease process

166. A 46-year-old man complained of back pain after doing spring planting in his garden. Two weeks later, upon examination by his doctor, it was noted that he had difficulty walking on his heels, and increased pain in the lower back, buttock, and dorsum of the foot on straight-leg raising to 30°. Deep tendon reflexes were normal. Which nerve root is involved?

    (A) L3
    (B) L4
    (C) L5
    (D) S1

167. A 25-year-old woman, who underwent an appendectomy 6 months ago, complains of a stabbing, colicky pain in the right lower abdomen. The pain is exacerbated by exercise and relieved by rest. It often radiates to the base of the labia and to the inner aspect of the thigh. Which of the following statements is likely to be true?

    (A) Surgical division of the nerve has caused severe neuralgia
    (B) The patient is suffering from entrapment of the genitofemoral nerve
    (C) An epidural steroid injection at L2–L3 may be helpful
    (D) The pain can be relieved by serial injections of local anesthetic, with or without steroids, injected at the point of maximum tenderness
    (E) The patient should have a pelvic MRI before any injections are done

Questions 168–169

A 76-year-old man complains of a 2-year history of progressive lower back pain with aching and numbness radiating from the right buttock to the lateral aspect and dorsum of his right foot. Pain is increased with walking. He found that he could walk with greater ease by leaning forward (i.e., leaning on a shopping cart and using it as support for ambulation). He is pain-free while supine.

168. What is the most likely diagnosis?

(A) Herniated nucleus pulposus
(B) Lumbar plexopathy
(C) Spinal stenosis
(D) Arachnoiditis

169. What electrodiagnostic finding would provide the most support for your diagnosis?

(A) Reduced amplitude of H-wave response
(B) Increased amplitude of the somatosensory evoked response
(C) Normal F-wave response
(D) Reduced conduction velocity of the genitofemoral nerve

---

170. All the following characteristics are commonly associated with postmastectomy pain syndrome EXCEPT

(A) the intercostobrachial nerve is often affected
(B) pain may be exacerbated by arm movement
(C) the patient complains of tight, constricting, burning pain in the midback
(D) painful areas often include the posterior arm and axilla
(E) patients may complain of pain in the anterior chest wall

171. Select the most appropriate statement regarding mucositis in cancer patients.

(A) Poor oral hygiene has no effect on the potential for development of mucositis
(B) Chemotherapy-induced mucositis usually begins 3 to 5 days after therapy is started
(C) There is no risk of an infection or hemorrhage associated with mucositis
(D) Radiation-induced mucositis appears 1 day after therapy is started
(E) Pain is characterized as mild in intensity and burning in quality

172. A 16-year-old boy who had an above-the-knee amputation complains of a painful, twisting, cramping sensation in his amputated calf, and pins and needles with burning in his amputated foot. The patient is suffering from

(A) stump pain
(B) reflex sympathetic dystrophy
(C) phantom limb pain
(D) Fabry's disease

173. A 5-year-old presents with a 2-year history of periumbilical pain, nausea, vomiting, headache, fever, and limb pains. The attacks last 4 to 5 h, resolve spontaneously, and recur four to five times per year. Multiple GI and fever work-ups are negative. Lead screening is also negative. The most likely diagnosis is

(A) appendicitis
(B) biliary colic
(C) lead intoxication
(D) abdominal migraine

174. A 50-year-old man presents with a 6-month history of weight loss, low-grade fever, fatigue, depression, and deep muscular aches of the neck, shoulder, and hip girdle, which are most severe in the morning or after exercise. No muscle tenderness or weakness is found on examination. What is the most likely diagnosis?

(A) Fibromyalgia
(B) Polymyalgia rheumatica
(C) Polymyositis
(D) Dermatomyositis

175. A 72-year-old man with a history of spinal stenosis has been a pain clinic patient for 2 years, receiving 4 to 6 months relief from epidural steroid injections before pain increases to the level where repeat injection is required. He presents to the clinic with the complaint of a recent increase in his pain. The pain is constant and is exacerbated by movement. It is not relieved by heat, NSAIDs, or bed rest. On examination, the patient is afebrile. The L4 and L5 vertebrae are tender to palpation. There is paraspinal muscle spasm. No motor or sensory deficits are present. The most likely diagnosis is

(A) vertebral osteomyelitis
(B) increasing spinal stenosis
(C) herniated disk
(D) Paget's disease

176. Postherpetic neuralgia is caused by

(A) herpes simplex type I
(B) herpes simplex type II
(C) varicella zoster
(D) Epstein-Barr virus

177. Which of the following is a Waddell's sign?

(A) The patient complains of back pain on dorsiflexion of the foot during straight-leg raising
(B) The patient complains of back pain during the skin roll test
(C) The patient demonstrates cogwheel movements of the back from flexion to standing upright
(D) There is absent rectal sphincter tone in the setting of low back pain

178. A 76-year-old woman complains of cramping pain in the low back and buttocks that radiates down the back of her thighs to her knees with prolonged standing or when she walks a short distance. She is able to walk more comfortably when she leans over a grocery cart to go food shopping, but complains of severe pain and paresthesias when she walks down small hills. This history is most suggestive of

(A) tabes dorsalis
(B) facet disease
(C) neurogenic claudication
(D) vascular claudication

179. A 20-year-old man complained of a severe, throbbing, bitemporal headache and facial flushing after eating a hot dog at the ball park. The headache and facial flushing subsided over the next few hours. The next week, the same event occurred. He commented on this to his physician at his annual physical. The doctor told him that he probably had

(A) hot dog headache
(B) sunburn from being in the bleachers
(C) food poisoning
(D) tension headache

180. A 50-year-old, previously healthy man presented to the emergency room with nausea, dizziness, and headache after eating at a Chinese restaurant. The symptoms subsided over the next several hours. Upon discharge from the emergency room, his physician told him to avoid which of the following?

(A) Nitrites
(B) Water chestnuts
(C) Monosodium glutamate
(D) Hot peppers

181. A 16-year-old girl with a history of childhood migraine saw her doctor with the complaint of intense midfrontal pain associated with eating frozen yogurt. The pain lasts 60 s before subsiding spontaneously. It happens almost every time she eats frozen yogurt. Which is the most likely diagnosis?

(A) Atypical migraine
(B) Temporomandibular joint syndrome
(C) Sinusitis
(D) Ice cream headache

182. An unpleasant abnormal sensation that is either evoked by a stimulus or occurs spontaneously without sensory stimulation is called

    (A) hyperpathia
    (B) paresthesia
    (C) hypoesthesia
    (D) dysesthesia

183. Pain in the left iliac region is frequently caused by all the following EXCEPT

    (A) acute salpingitis
    (B) twisted ovarian cyst
    (C) ulcerative colitis
    (D) acute diverticulitis
    (E) Meckel's diverticulitis

184. Pain from visceral structures in the abdomen can be caused by all the following EXCEPT

    (A) inflammation
    (B) crush injury
    (C) overdistention
    (D) traction
    (E) ischemia

185. Patrick's sign is present most frequently in patients who have

    (A) sciatica
    (B) herniated disk
    (C) hip joint disease
    (D) facet syndrome

186. A 35-year-old man with a 20-year history of spondylolysis of L5 after a football injury develops acute pain in the buttocks and upper posterior thigh. Severe spasm of the hamstrings causes him to walk with a shuffling gait. The most likely cause of his acute symptoms is

    (A) facet syndrome
    (B) herniated disk
    (C) sacroiliitis
    (D) spondylolisthesis

Questions 187–189

A patient is unable to push the examiner's hand away when the arm is flexed at the elbow.

187. The major muscle involved in this action is

    (A) biceps
    (B) deltoid
    (C) triceps
    (D) brachioradialis

188. The primary innervation of the muscles that allow extension of the forearm is from which nerve?

    (A) Radial
    (B) Musculocutaneous
    (C) Ulnar
    (D) Median

189. The patient was found to have a herniated disk on MRI. Disk herniation at which level would be most likely to produce weakness on attempting to extend the forearm against resistance?

    (A) C3–C4
    (B) C6–C7
    (C) C7–T1
    (D) T1–T2

190. The most common vertebral level at which fracture of the pars interarticularis occurs is

    (A) L2
    (B) L3
    (C) L4
    (D) L5

191. A 20-year-old woman complains of a long history of episodic, generalized, colicky, abdominal pain and nausea whose episodes resolve in 1 to 3 days. The pain occurs most frequently during her menses or when she is emotionally upset. Multiple medical evaluations and exploratory laparotomies have not revealed the cause of her problem. Abdominal radiographs show a thumbprinting pattern of the small bowel. The most likely diagnosis is

    (A) endometriosis
    (B) acute intermittent porphyria
    (C) hereditary angioedema
    (D) eosinophilic enteritis

192. A 27-year-old man with ankylosing spondylitis complains of neck, occipital, and shoulder pain. He denies any history of recent trauma or febrile illness. The most likely cause of his pain is

    (A) compression fracture of C2
    (B) cervical osteomyelitis
    (C) atlantoaxial subluxation
    (D) epidural hematoma

193. A 22-year-old man complains of a severely aching and throbbing, unilateral headache associated with mydriasis and hyperhidrosis of the painful side. The headaches last 12 to 24 h before subsiding. A CT scan of the brain shows nothing abnormal. He has a history of a knife wound to the neck 1 year ago. The most likely diagnosis is posttraumatic

    (A) dysautonomic cephalgia
    (B) cluster headache
    (C) muscle contraction headache
    (D) basilar artery migraine

194. A 45-year-old woman with systemic lupus erythematosus complains of fever, headache, and vomiting associated with a depressed level of consciousness over the last 24 h. She recently had begun taking ibuprofen as treatment for diffuse joint pain. CSF examination revealed neutrophilia and normal glucose. The most likely diagnosis is

    (A) bacterial meningitis
    (B) drug-induced meningitis
    (C) fungal meningitis
    (D) viral meningitis

195. A 44-year-old woman complains of intense, throbbing, bitemporal headache that occurs 4 to 6 h after she exercises and resolves with 1 dose of 400 to 600 mg of ibuprofen. What is the most likely diagnosis?

    (A) Brain tumor
    (B) Pheochromocytoma
    (C) Multiple sclerosis
    (D) Exertional headache

196. A 10-year-old boy complains of upper neck and jaw pain that has persisted since his tonsillectomy 6 months ago. The pain is intensified by swallowing, talking, or turning his head. He is afebrile and blood work shows no evidence of infection. Which of the following is the most likely cause of his persistent pain?

    (A) Riedel's struma
    (B) Eagle's syndrome
    (C) Ludwig's angina
    (D) Posttraumatic stress disorder

197. Ninety percent of cervical radiculopathies caused by disk impingement involve which nerve roots?

    (A) C3, C4
    (B) C4, C5
    (C) C5, C6
    (D) C6, C7

198. A patient complains of shoulder and proximal arm pain. There is weakness of abduction (deltoid) and loss of the biceps reflex. The patient denies hand pain. Sensory examination is normal. The cervical MRI reveals the impingement of a disk upon a nerve root. What is the most likely level of the lesion?

(A) C4
(B) C5
(C) C6
(D) C7

199. A 41-year-old man complains of pain involving his neck, shoulders, posterolateral arm, and hand, which occurred after a strenuous upper body workout with weights. He has also noted numbness and paresthesias in his index and middle fingers. On examination, there is marked weakness of the triceps and extensor carpi radialis and ulnaris. The triceps reflex is absent. The most likely nerve root involved is

(A) C5
(B) C6
(C) C7
(D) C8

200. A patient complains of pain involving the entire arm as well as numbness and tingling in the thumb and index finger. On examination, there is marked weakness of the biceps and brachialis muscles. Both the biceps and brachioradialis reflexes are abnormal. A lesion of which nerve root is most likely to produce these symptoms and signs?

(A) C5
(B) C6
(C) C7
(D) C8

201. A patient has pain in the medial side of the arm and forearm that radiates into the ring and little fingers and is associated with normal reflexes and weakness of the intrinsic muscles of the hand. This indicates a lesion of which cervical nerve root?

(A) C5
(B) C6
(C) C7
(D) C8

202. The most common cause of an epidural abscess is

(A) *Staphylococcus aureus*
(B) *Pseudomonas* species
(C) gram-negative rods
(D) streptococcal species

203. Torticollis may be caused by all the following EXCEPT

(A) herniated cervical disk
(B) ingestion of phenothiazine
(C) injection of botulinum toxin
(D) syringomyelia

204. A 62-year-old man complains of a 6-month history of unilateral, constant neck and occipital pain associated with numbness in the back of his head, which occurred after he was "rear-ended" in a motor vehicle accident. The most likely diagnosis is

(A) malingering
(B) occipital migraine
(C) occipital neuralgia
(D) cervical disk herniation

205. A 36-year-old secretary complained for 4 months of paresthesias and aching in the right hand, especially notable after typing for several hours. The aching and numbness were most pronounced in the middle finger and medial aspect of her forearm. The aching, tingling, and numbness made it difficult for her to sleep at night. She also noted some weakness in right grip strength. What is the most likely diagnosis?

(A) Pancoast syndrome
(B) Ulnar neuropathy
(C) Radial nerve entrapment
(D) Carpal tunnel syndrome
(E) Reflex sympathetic dystrophy

206. A 56-year-old woman with breast cancer complains of pain and tenderness of her muscles and joints that began 24 h after she began a taper-off of prednisone. She is afebrile. Blood work does not reveal any significant abnormalities. Bone scan does not reveal new metastases. What is the most likely cause of her symptoms?

(A) Anxiety
(B) Viral influenza
(C) Steroid pseudorheumatism
(D) Arthritis

207. Geniculate neuralgia is
    (A) most often seen in elderly patients
    (B) called the Ramsay Hunt syndrome when accompanied by ipsilateral facial paralysis
    (C) associated with ocular pain
    (D) more common than glossopharyngeal neuralgia

208. A 67-year-old man with persistent paresis on the left side and who had a cerebrovascular accident 6 months ago began to notice a burning, aching, and occasionally shooting pain on his affected side. Full neurologic evaluation did not reveal new injuries. The most likely cause of his pain is
    (A) cancer
    (B) reflex sympathetic dystrophy
    (C) conversion reaction
    (D) central poststroke pain syndrome

209. Select the true statement from the following.
    (A) Syringomyelia is common after trauma to the spinal cord
    (B) Pain is common in syringomyelia
    (C) Patients with syringomyelia commonly have normal temperature sensibility
    (D) Syringomyelia is commonly treated by spinal cord stimulation

210. All the following statements are true regarding the occurrence of acute herpes zoster (AHZ) in cancer patients EXCEPT
    (A) patients with hematologic or lymphoproliferative cancer have an increased incidence of AHZ
    (B) the location of the AHZ infection is not associated with the site of the cancer
    (C) patients receiving immunosuppressive therapies have an increased incidence of AHZ
    (D) AHZ occurs less frequently in nonirradiated areas than in irradiated areas

211. A 52-year-old man complains of a sudden onset of severe, stabbing pain in the left jaw and cheek that subsides in less than a minute. He is pain-free during the intervals between attacks. Activities such as combing his hair and shaving can cause the onset of his facial pain. He is otherwise healthy. The most likely diagnosis is
    (A) atypical facial pain
    (B) vascular facial pain
    (C) trigeminal neuralgia
    (D) postherpetic neuralgia

212. Painful polyneuropathies caused by selective small fiber loss include all the following EXCEPT
    (A) chronic renal failure
    (B) diabetes
    (C) amyloid neuropathy
    (D) hereditary sensory neuropathy
    (E) Fabry's disease

213. Painful polyneuropathies with selective loss of large fibers include all the following EXCEPT
    (A) diabetic neuropathy
    (B) isoniazid neuropathy
    (C) pellagra neuropathy
    (D) hypothyroid neuropathy

214. A 3-year-old, mildly retarded boy is brought in to the ER for treatment of a tongue laceration. His mother gives a history of multiple episodes in which he accidentally injured himself without seeming to feel any pain. She states that he has burnt his hands several times picking up hot objects without obvious discomfort. He also has been to the hospital many times for evaluation of high fevers. His clinical presentation suggests
    (A) trisomy 21
    (B) congenital analgesia
    (C) child abuse
    (D) lead poisoning

Questions 215–216

A 56-year-old woman, who has undergone two spinal surgeries, complains of persistent, gradually worsening, burning, and lancinating pain in the right buttock radiating down the lateral thigh to the middorsum of the right foot. MRI shows patent neural foramina and adequate spinal alignment. There is clustering of the lumbar nerve roots with adherence to the meninges in the right side of the spinal canal.

215. The most likely diagnosis is

   (A) herniated nucleus pulposus
   (B) malingering
   (C) fractured pars interarticularis
   (D) arachnoiditis
   (E) spondylolisthesis

216. Appropriate therapies for this patient would include all the following EXCEPT

   (A) spinal cord stimulation
   (B) physical therapy
   (C) piroxicam
   (D) intrathecal steroids
   (E) carbamazepine

---

217. True statements regarding posttraumatic headache include that it

   (A) can follow even mild head injury
   (B) is not usually associated with personality changes
   (C) causes bilateral ocular pain
   (D) is associated with conjunctival injection and rhinorrhea
   (E) is best treated with oxygen

218. A 63-year-old woman complains of recent onset of unilateral temporal headaches. She has muscle and joint aches without neck stiffness. She also complains of loss of appetite, low-grade fever, and visual disturbances. The most likely diagnosis is

   (A) migraine headaches
   (B) subarachnoid hemorrhage
   (C) viral influenza
   (D) giant cell arteritis
   (E) venous thrombosis

219. All the conditions listed can cause referred pain to the coccyx EXCEPT

   (A) levator syndrome
   (B) arachnoiditis
   (C) pilonidal cyst
   (D) fracture of the L3 vertebral body
   (E) vaginismus

220. A 25-year-old, obese man complains of a burning pain in the anterolateral thigh. Deep tendon reflexes and findings in a motor examination are normal. There is a slight sensory deficit in the lateral thigh that corresponds to the painful area. What is the most appropriate diagnostic block to perform on this patient?

   (A) Epidural local anesthetic and steroid
   (B) Trigger point injection
   (C) Ilioinguinal nerve block
   (D) Lumbar sympathetic block
   (E) Lateral femoral cutaneous nerve block

221. A 32-year-old man complains of a 2-week history of a deep, steady, dull headache localized to his left occiput and upper neck. The headache is intermittent. It does not interfere with sleep, but seems worse on awakening. The headache worsens with coughing. Acetaminophen and ibuprofen relieve the headache. However, it recurs after the analgesic wears off. The patient denies prior history of headaches or history of head trauma. The most likely diagnosis is

   (A) migraine headache
   (B) cluster headache
   (C) frontal lobe tumor
   (D) posterior fossa tumor
   (E) Tolosa-Hunt syndrome

Questions 222–223

A 13-year-old girl presents with recent onset of cramping abdominal pain associated with occasional vomiting and low-grade fever. She is also found to have postural hypotension and diminishing upper and lower extremity deep tendon reflexes with paresthesias of her feet and hands. She has recently been having difficulty with schoolwork.

222. What is the most likely diagnosis?

(A) Hyperventilation syndrome
(B) Anorexia nervosa
(C) Appendicitis
(D) Acute intermittent porphyria

223. The diagnosis can be confirmed by

(A) exploratory laparotomy
(B) complete blood count with differential
(C) 24-h urine collection
(D) arterial blood gas

---

224. Which of the following activities places the greatest load on the L3 disk in a 70-kg person?

(A) Bending forward 20°
(B) Bending sideways
(C) Lifting 20 kg, back bent, knees straight
(D) Lifting 20 kg, back straight, knees bent

225. The sitting position that places the lowest load on the L3 disk is with the back of the chair at

(A) 90° without a lumbar support cushion
(B) 90° with a lumbar support cushion
(C) 110° without lumbar support
(D) 100° with lumbar support

226. Which of the following statements is true regarding sickle cell disease?

(A) Valine is substituted for glutamic acid in the sixth acid of the beta chain of hemoglobin
(B) With proper treatment, patients with homozygous sickle cell disease have a normal life expectancy
(C) Splenectomy and hematinics have been shown to be effective in prolonging life expectancy and decreasing frequency of crises in patients with severe sickle cell disease
(D) Homozygous patients have mostly HbS, less HbA, and a small amount of HbF

227. A 21-year-old, male dock worker complains of a 6-month history of an aching right arm, which is exacerbated by carrying heavy objects or by raising his arms over his head. On physical examination, a fullness of the supraclavicular fossa is noted. No neurologic deficits were found. There was obliteration of the radial pulse with arm extension and abduction. What is the most likely diagnosis?

(A) Pancoast's tumor
(B) Brachial plexitis
(C) Neurofibroma of the brachial plexus
(D) Thoracic outlet syndrome
(E) Herniated nucleus pulposus

228. In order of most to least frequent, the divisions of the trigeminal nerve involved in tic douloureux are

(A) V1, V2, V3
(B) V1, V3, V2
(C) V2, V3, V1
(D) V3, V1, V2

229. True statements regarding the stress response to injury include all the following EXCEPT

   (A) it is a complex hormonal and neurologic response
   (B) it is mediated via sympathetic pathways
   (C) a catabolic response predominates
   (D) hypoglycemia is typically observed
   (E) serum aldosterone levels are elevated

230. A 61-year-old woman presents to the pain clinic with a chief complaint of left shoulder and arm pain 3 years after undergoing radiation therapy for breast cancer. Physical examination reveals lymphedema of the left axilla with noticeable skin changes. Examination of the left supraclavicular area precipitates a sharp pain that radiates down her left arm. Which of the following is her likely diagnosis?

   (A) Cervical radiculopathy
   (B) Tumor metastasis
   (C) Reflex sympathetic dystrophy
   (D) Radiation-induced plexopathy
   (E) Thrombangiitis obliterans

231. A 26-year-old man complains of a painful scrotum. The patient should undergo careful evaluation for all the following conditions EXCEPT

   (A) testicular torsion
   (B) epididymo-orchitis
   (C) testicular cancer
   (D) paraphimosis
   (E) fractured testicle

232. Which of the following series of tests and procedures would be most helpful in distinguishing testicular torsion from epididymo-orchitis?

   (A) Urinalysis, ice with elevation and immobilization, needle aspiration
   (B) Urinalysis, radioactive testicular scan, ultrasound, surgical exploration
   (C) Urinalysis, ultrasound, testicular biopsy
   (D) Urinalysis, ultrasound, needle aspiration, testicular biopsy
   (E) Urinalysis, ultrasound, ice with elevation and immobilization, surgical exploration

233. A patient with right foot reflex sympathetic dystrophy has responded well to a series of lumbar sympathetic blocks. What advice would you give her to prevent it from recurring?

   (A) Minimize walking
   (B) Minimize any weight bearing on the foot
   (C) Wear a protective boot whenever possible walking or weight bearing
   (D) Wear comfortable, supportive shoes while maintaining normal physical activity and take care not to reinjure the foot

234. Which of the following activities will exacerbate pain the most in an elderly patient with severe spinal stenosis?

   (A) Walking uphill
   (B) Walking downhill
   (C) Riding a bicycle
   (D) Bending forward

235. More than 80 percent of patients with clinically apparent reflex sympathetic dystrophy will have positive

   (A) blood pool images
   (B) radionuclide angiograms
   (C) early phase bone scans
   (D) delayed image bone scans

236. Which nerve is entrapped at the wrist in carpal tunnel syndrome?

   (A) Radial
   (B) Median
   (C) Ulnar
   (D) Musculocutaneous
   (E) Anterior interosseus

237. A 32-year-old, HIV-positive man complains of painful burning soles of both feet. What is the most likely explanation for this pain?

   (A) Secondary infection with herpes zoster
   (B) Guillain-Barré syndrome
   (C) Acute psychosis
   (D) HIV-related sensory neuropathy
   (E) HIV encephalopathy

DIRECTIONS: Each question below contains four suggested responses of which **one or more** is correct. Select

A	if	**1, 2, and 3**	are correct
B	if	**1 and 3**	are correct
C	if	**2 and 4**	are correct
D	if	**4**	is correct
E	if	**1, 2, 3, and 4**	are correct

238. True statements regarding Eagle's syndrome include which of the following?

    (1) Trigger points are present
    (2) Pain occurs during mandibular movement or twisting of the neck
    (3) Pain can occur spontaneously with the mouth closed
    (4) The pain is stabbing in nature

239. Which of the following would support the diagnosis of an S1 nerve root lesion?

    (1) Absent ankle jerk
    (2) Weakness in toe walking
    (3) Atrophy of the gastrocnemius
    (4) Knee pain

240. True statements regarding drug therapy in terminal pain syndromes include

    (1) anxiolytics are useful
    (2) anti-inflammatory agents are useful
    (3) narcotics are useful
    (4) neural blockade is not useful

241. Correct statements regarding chronic pain include that it

    (1) is not biologically useful
    (2) has poorly defined peripheral mechanisms
    (3) has poorly defined central pathways
    (4) involves the physiologic stress response

242. True statements regarding deafferentation pain syndromes include that they

    (1) are rarely successfully treated with narcotic agents
    (2) may manifest as burning, crushing, or tearing pain
    (3) typically produce pain that is constant and unremitting
    (4) commonly respond to neurosurgical intervention

243. Characteristic features of peripheral neuropathies include

    (1) paresthesias and dysesthesias
    (2) sensory loss
    (3) loss or diminution of tendon reflexes
    (4) pain

244. True statements regarding pathophysiologic factors of terminal pain include

    (1) it is not biologically harmful
    (2) there is well-defined tissue damage
    (3) it is a variant of chronic pain
    (4) the stress response is harmful

245. Positive Waddell's signs are indicative of

    (1) the effects of psychosocial factors
    (2) a positive response to surgical intervention
    (3) need for a comprehensive evaluation of pain
    (4) facet joint arthropathy

246. All the following statements correctly differentiate chronic paroxysmal hemicrania (CPH) from cluster headaches EXCEPT

    (1) attacks of CPH last for longer periods of time
    (2) episodes of CPH are more frequent
    (3) CPH occurs more commonly at night
    (4) CPH can be effectively treated with indomethacin

247. Several painful conditions have been described in patients with AIDS. These include

    (1) Guillain-Barré syndrome
    (2) postherpetic neuralgia
    (3) encephalopathy
    (4) predominant sensory neuropathy

SUMMARY OF DIRECTIONS				
A	B	C	D	E
1,2,3 only	1,3 only	2,4 only	4 only	All are correct

248. Increases in plasma concentration of alpha-1-acid glycoprotein have been associated with
    (1) patients with cancer
    (2) patients with chronic pain
    (3) patients who have had myocardial infarction
    (4) neonates

249. Painful conditions associated with nonselective neural fiber loss include
    (1) myeloma
    (2) Fabry's disease
    (3) alcoholic neuropathy
    (4) Tangier disease

250. Which of the following signs may be associated with T1 root compression?
    (1) Weakness of the intrinsic muscles of the hand
    (2) Subjective numbness in the ulnar aspect of the forearm
    (3) Pain in the neck, medial scapula, and anterior chest
    (4) Horner's syndrome

251. Which of the following can be associated with a neuropathic pain syndrome?
    (1) Diabetes
    (2) Mercury poisoning
    (3) Causalgia
    (4) Guillain-Barré syndrome

252. Examples of neuropathic pain syndromes include
    (1) phantom limb pain
    (2) dyspareunia
    (3) thalamic syndrome
    (4) vaginismus

253. True statements regarding the use of ketamine in trauma patients include
    (1) it may be used as the sole agent for trauma surgery
    (2) it possesses sympathomimetic action
    (3) at lower doses it is an analgesic
    (4) it can be used in trauma patients with head injuries

254. Diagnostic features of an epidural abscess include that it
    (1) is most commonly caused by *Staphylococcus epidermidis*
    (2) may present as severe back pain
    (3) will show normal myelographic findings
    (4) may present as local back tenderness

255. True statements regarding glossopharyngeal neuralgia include
    (1) it is more common in adults than children
    (2) attacks can be associated with cardiac arrest
    (3) it is most often described as aching and burning between attacks
    (4) it is found to occur more frequently in patients with tic douloureux

256. True statements regarding central pain in spinal cord injury (SCI) include which of the following?
    (1) Few SCI patients complain of moderate to severe central pain
    (2) Many SCI patients suffer from visceral pain
    (3) Spinal cord stimulation is a highly effective treatment for most SCI-associated pain
    (4) Dorsal root entry zone (DREZ) lesions have been tried with varying success as treatment for SCI-associated pain

TYPES OF PAIN

257. True statements regarding Parkinson's disease include which of the following?

(1) A significant proportion of patients with Parkinson's disease complain of pain, tingling, and numbness
(2) Most of the pain associated with Parkinson's disease is related to fluctuations in motor symptoms
(3) Proper adjustment of antiparkinsonian medications often decreases pain symptoms
(4) Droperidol has been used to decrease the pain related to Parkinson's disease

258. Headache types more common in women include

(1) tension headache
(2) giant cell arteritis
(3) migraine headache
(4) cluster headache

259. Phantom limb sensation is described by which of the following?

(1) It is a very common occurrence in the first month after amputation
(2) It is strongest in below-knee amputations
(3) It occurs more frequently in older amputee patients
(4) It is weakest in above-elbow amputations

260. In the evaluation of a patient complaining of testicular pain, which of the following diagnostic tests would be helpful in establishing a diagnosis?

(1) Urinalysis
(2) Testicular biopsy
(3) Testicular ultrasound
(4) Radioactive testicular scans

261. Referred pain to the penis can be caused by which of the following neuralgias?

(1) Ilioinguinal
(2) Iliohypogastric
(3) Genitofemoral
(4) Lateral femoral cutaneous

262. Treatment of Reiter's syndrome may include

(1) NSAIDS
(2) azathioprine
(3) methotrexate
(4) plasmapheresis

263. Which of the following conditions can be associated with a painful peripheral neuropathy?

(1) AIDS
(2) Sjögren's syndrome
(3) Guillain-Barré syndrome
(4) Insulinoma

264. Priapism is a prolonged, painful penile erection that is

(1) seen in patients with leukemia
(2) an emergency condition
(3) a potential cause of erectile impotence
(4) seen in patients with sickle cell disease

265. A 27-year-old runner developed a 2nd metatarsal stress fracture. Four months later, she developed temperature changes, swelling, and burning pain in her foot. What diagnostic tests or procedures may be helpful in establishing a diagnosis?

(1) Delayed image bone scans
(2) Plain film of the foot
(3) Lumbar sympathetic block
(4) Intravenous lidocaine

266. Which of the following should be present to make the diagnosis of acute radicular syndrome?

(1) Leg pain as the dominant complaint when compared with back pain
(2) Neurologic symptoms in a typical dermatomal distribution
(3) Significant straight-leg raising findings
(4) Evidence of disk herniation on MRI

267. Characteristics of Raeder's syndrome (paratrigeminal neuralgia) include

(1) frontotemporal pain
(2) amaurosis fugax
(3) incomplete Horner's syndrome
(4) transient facial paralysis

268. The differential diagnosis for occipital neuralgia should include

(1) whiplash
(2) metastatic neoplasm at the base of the skull
(3) herniated cervical intervertebral disk
(4) cluster headache

SUMMARY OF DIRECTIONS				
A	B	C	D	E
1,2,3 only	1,3 only	2,4 only	4 only	All are correct

269. Which of the following should be present to make the diagnosis of temporomandibular pain and dysfunction syndrome?

   (1) Pain and tenderness of the masticatory muscles
   (2) Joint sounds with jaw opening
   (3) Limited mandibular movement
   (4) History of bruxism

270. Conditions that increase the risk of developing carpal tunnel syndrome include

   (1) pregnancy
   (2) rheumatoid arthritis
   (3) gout
   (4) amyloidosis

Types of Pain

Answers

146. **The answer is D.** (*Ready, p 2.*) Pain is defined as an unpleasant sensory and emotional experience associated with actual or potential tissue damage or described in terms of such damage. Suffering is the reaction of an organism to the experience of pain. Nociception is the process of detecting and signaling the presence of a noxious stimulus. A noxious stimulus is one of an intensity that is damaging or potentially damaging to the integrity of tissue.

147. **The answer is A.** (*Wall, p 715.*) C5 nerve root compression is associated with pain in the neck, shoulder, medial scapula, anterior chest, and lateral aspect of the upper arm. Weakness of the deltoid, supraspinatus, infraspinatus, biceps, and brachioradialis, with diminished biceps and brachioradialis deep tendon reflexes, may also be present.

148. **The answer is B.** (*Wall, p 715.*) The patient has evidence of C6 root compression, most likely due to C5-C6 disk protrusion. Pain in the neck, shoulder, medial scapula, anterior chest, lateral aspect of the upper arm, and dorsal aspect of the forearm associated with biceps and extensor carpi radialis weakness is frequently present. The patient may complain of numbness of the thumb and index finger. The biceps reflex may be diminished or absent.

149. **The answer is C.** (*Wall, p 882.*) Allodynia is the perception of pain produced by stimuli that are usually nonpainful. Hyperalgesia is hypersensitivity to noxious stimuli. Patients who suffer from central pain, neuropathic pain, and sympathetically maintained pain have a high incidence of allodynia and hyperalgesia.

150. **The answer is A.** (*Raj, p 76.*) From easiest to most difficult to treat, the types of pain are ranked as follows:

    Continuous somatic pain
    Intermittent somatic pain
    Continuous visceral pain
    Intermittent visceral pain
    Continuous neuropathic pain
    Intermittent neuropathic pain
    Chronic pain
    Psychogenic pain

151. **The answer is D.** (*Raj, p 877.*) Any stimulus that damages or deforms tissue sufficiently to activate somatic or visceral nociceptive terminals causes the conscious experience of pain. The unpleasant sensations of lacerations, contusions, fractures, inflammation, distended viscera, and tissue invasion by cancer are all examples of nociceptive pain. Phantom limb pain is an example of a deafferentation pain syndrome.

PAIN MANAGEMENT

152. The answer is A. (*Raj, pp 877–880.*) Patients with nociceptive pain often describe it as intermittent, cramping, aching, throbbing, or, alternatively, sharp or shooting in nature. Changes in position or activity level may improve or worsen the pain. Narcotic analgesics relieve nociceptive pain, as does local anesthetic blockade.

153. The answer is C. (*Raj, pp 272–273.*) Pain in the posterior aspect of the arm is likely due to a C7 root lesion, whereas medial anterior or lateral arm pain may be due to C6 or C7 nerve root lesions. A C7 nerve root lesion will also produce symptoms (pain and paresthesias) in the index and middle fingers as well as a diminished or absent triceps reflex. Absence of a brachioradialis reflex is an indication of a C6 nerve root lesion.

154. The answer is B. (*Raj, p 67.*) There are significant clinical differences between visceral and cutaneous nociception. There are fewer nociceptors in the viscera than in the skin, and these receptors may have a different activation profile. Cutting and burning of mesentery, the uterine cervix, or other visceral organs do not necessarily produce clinical pain. However, traction, distention, or ischemia will produce a type of pain. This pain is often diffuse and poorly localized and often has a significant autonomic component. The visceral nociceptors have wide receptive fields that prevent accurate localization of visceral sensation, which may explain the phenomenon of referred pain.

155. The answer is D. (*Raj, p 236.*) Ramsay Hunt syndrome develops from a herpes zoster infection involving the geniculate ganglion. Zoster lesions of the external ear and oral mucosa on the ipsilateral side are usually observed. The syndrome can present as a deep, painful sensation primarily behind the ear between the pinna and mastoid process and radiating to the face, ear, neck, and occipital areas.

156. The answer is E. (*Wall, pp 510–511.*) Diagnostic criteria for temporal arteritis (giant cell arteritis) include the presence of typical histopathologic features on temporal artery biopsy, a swollen and tender scalp artery, elevated ESR, and the disappearance of the headache with 48 h of steroid therapy. The headache is usually temporal, of variable severity, having a constant, boring quality, and is temporarily relieved by analgesics such as aspirin. Polymyalgia rheumatica as well as general malaise, anorexia, or mild fever frequently accompanies this systemic disease.

157. The answer is A. (*Bonica, p 1301.*) Endometriosis can cause pain and tenderness by direct action on nerve endings or by interfering with the function of involved or adjacent organs. The pain is characteristically worse a few days before menstruation rather than during the early period of flow. Hypogastric midcycle pain (mittelschmerz) in patients with endometriosis can be severe for a few hours to days and can mimic the pain of acute appendicitis.

158. The answer is B. (*Raj, p 237.*) Sluder's neuralgia, also known as sphenopalatine ganglion neuralgia, is an uncommon facial neuralgia characterized by severe pain in the face below the eyebrows. The pain is unilateral, constant, and boring. The cause of Sluder's syndrome is thought to be involvement of the sphenopalatine ganglion from an irritation such as sinusitis.

159. The answer is C. (*Wall, p 506.*) A single attack of cluster headache can be successfully treated with inhalation of 100% oxygen in 60 to 70 percent of cases. Other possible treatments for cluster headache include intranasal application of dihydroergotamine and intramuscular sumatriptan, which is an agonist of 5-HTD receptors.

160. The answer is E. (*Raj, p 777.*) The cause of an epidural abscess is usually hematogenous, particularly from a source in the pelvis, and is only rarely introduced from outside the body. The most common symptom is pain in the back, which progresses to radicular pain with sensory and motor disturbances. It can progress rapidly to paraplegia unless the diagnosis is made. The onset is usually a few days, but may take up to 2 weeks in some cases.

161. The answer is A. (*Raj, p 207.*) Tension headache usually occurs bilaterally but can be unilateral, often involving the frontal, temporal, and occipital regions. These headaches evolve over a period of hours to days and then tend to remain constant without progressive symptoms. Significant sleep disturbance is present in most sufferers of tension headaches. Although both sexes are affected, females predominate. There is no hereditary pattern to tension headache, but it may occur in family clusters as children mimic and learn the pain behavior of their parents.

162. The answer is C. (*Raj, p 518.*) Acute herpes zoster lesions appear in the thoracic dermatomes in more than 50 percent of patients. The next region most commonly involved is the trigeminal distribution (3 to 20 percent); the ophthalmic division is involved in 75 percent of these patients. Lumbar and cervical eruptions occur in 10 to 20 percent of patients. A sacral distribution is much less common.

163. The answer is A. (*Raj, p 114.*) The straight-leg raising test (Lasègue's sign) is most significant if it reproduces the patient's pain in the low back, buttocks, or leg. If pain occurs at less than 40°, it is indicative of a disk protrusion against a nerve root. If straight-leg raising on the opposite side produces pain in the affected limb, this further supports the diagnosis of a herniated disk. If pain occurs on the straight-leg raising test of the affected limb at 70 to 80°, this indicates a sensitive nerve root, but not necessarily a disk protrusion.

164. The answer is D. (*Wall, p 674.*) The patient has symptoms consistent with Guillain-Barré acute inflammatory demyelinating polyneuropathy. Pain is a common early symptom of the disease. The patient may complain of muscular or radicular pain or both, followed by sensorimotor dysfunction. The pain may be severe but usually resolves as the symptoms improve.

165. The answer is D. (*Wall, p 893.*) Multiple sclerosis (MS) is a neuroinflammatory disease associated with the destruction of myelin, axons, and cell bodies in the CNS. Pain is a problem for many patients with MS. Central pain is the most common type. Though the incidence of trigeminal neuralgia is higher in MS patients than in the general population, its incidence is significantly lower than that of generalized central pain in MS patients. Patients may also suffer from musculoskeletal pain, peripheral neurogenic pain, and, rarely, primary psychogenic pain. The incidence of headaches is not increased in MS patients.

166. The answer is C. (*Wall, p 717.*) L5 root compression may cause pain in the low back, buttock, posterolateral thigh, lateral aspect of the lower leg, lateral malleolus, dorsum of the foot, and occasionally in the groin. Numbness of the dorsum of the foot, big toe, and lateral aspect of the lower leg and weakness of the tibialis anterior, extensor hallucis longus, extensor digitorum brevis, and sometimes the gluteal muscles may occur. Occasionally, the biceps femoris reflex will be diminished, though on most examinations of deep tendon reflexes no significant abnormalities would be found. In this patient, the exacerbation of pain on straight-leg raising to 30° would suggest L5 root compression due to a disk (usually L4–L5) protrusion.

167. The answer is D. (*Wall, p 608.*) The patient is suffering from entrapment of the ilioinguinal nerve (L1–L2), which innervates the muscles of the lower abdomen, the skin over the inguinal ligament, the base of the labia, and the inner aspect of the thigh. The nerve becomes superficial just medial to the anterior superior iliac spine. The pain is stabbing and colicky and worsens with exercise. Treatment consists of serial injections of local anesthetic with or without steroid over the site of maximum tenderness. If this is unsuccessful, surgical division of the nerve can be considered.

168–169. The answers are 168-C, 169-A. (*Bonica, p 635.*) The patient has lumbar spinal stenosis involving the L5 and S1 nerve roots most prominently. Spinal stenosis is a slowly progressive disease and therefore allows for neural adaptation over time. Slowing of nerve conduction velocity occurs through the region of neurologic impairment. Needle EMG may not show evidence of membrane instability. Motor unit action potentials may have increased amplitude and duration because of collateral reinnervation, which occurs over time. Somatosensory evoked potentials will be abnormal to varying degrees in the dermatomes of the affected nerve roots. Both F- and H-wave late responses will be abnormal.

170. **The answer is C.** (*Jacox, p 34.*) The patient with postmastectomy pain may complain of a tight, constricting, burning pain in the posterior arm, axilla, and anterior chest wall, with the pain being exacerbated by movement of the arm. The intercostobrachial nerve is often affected. Patients may respond to a combination of therapies, including stellate ganglion blocks, thoracic epidural blocks, transcutaneous electrical nerve stimulation (TENS), anticonvulsants, and other medications used to treat neuropathic pain.

171. **The answer is B.** (*Jacox, p 38.*) Mucositis may be a complication of chemotherapy or radiation therapy to the head and neck. There may be an increased risk in patients with poor oral hygiene. Pain is intense. Swallowing may be intolerable and oral intake may need to be restricted. Mucosal thickening, sloughing, ulceration, and fibrous exudate occur. In chemotherapy-induced mucositis, pain usually begins 3 to 5 days after the initial dose and peaks in 7 to 10 days, with slow resolution over the next week. Complications such as secondary infection or hemorrhage can occur. In radiation-induced mucositis, the symptoms usually begin the second week of treatment, peak the fourth week, and may persist for 2 to 3 weeks after therapy is completed. Treatment may be topical (local anesthetics/capsaicin) or systemic (e.g., IV patient-controlled anesthesia [PCA]).

172. **The answer is C.** (*Bonica, pp 244–246.*) Phantom limb sensation is very common in patients after amputation. Patients will often complain of the sensation that the amputated limb is still present, though it may be distorted in position or length. "Telescoping" of the phantom sensation occurs over time, until it resolves in about 1 year in most patients. While the majority of patients experience phantom limb sensation, a smaller number complain of phantom limb pain.

173. **The answer is D.** (*Bonica, p 1271.*) Abdominal migraine occurs mostly in children between the ages of 3 and 10. There is an increased incidence in children who suffer from migraine headaches and also in children who have relatives who suffer from migraine. A large percentage of children who suffer from abdominal migraine will progress to migraine headaches as adults. The symptom complex consists of recurrent and identical attacks of periumbilical pain, nausea, vomiting, headache, pallor, perspiration, bradycardia, fever, diarrhea, and limb pains lasting less than 6 h. The children are symptom-free between attacks. Appendicitis, biliary colic, pancreatitis, gallbladder disease, lead intoxication, and any other abdominal process must be ruled out. If ergotamine is given and the attacks decrease or are eliminated, the diagnosis of abdominal migraine is confirmed.

174. **The answer is B.** (*Bonica, pp 388–392.*) Polymyalgia rheumatica is a painful condition in which patients complain of deep muscular aching beginning in the neck, shoulder, and hip girdle. Stiffness is most severe in the morning and after activity. Patients may complain of malaise, low-grade fever, depression, fatigue, and weight loss. There is no muscle tenderness or weakness. Sedimentation rate is markedly elevated, and an associated arteritis may result in blindness. Treatment consists of oral steroid therapy and nonnarcotic analgesics. Fibromyalgia is associated with multiple tender points and muscle stiffness. Polymyositis and dermatomyositis are associated with proximal muscle weakness of the limbs and muscles, which are tender on palpation.

175. **The answer is A.** (*Bonica, pp 393–394.*) The symptoms described in the question are consistent with the diagnosis of vertebral osteomyelitis. Clinical features include persistent, localized pain with heat, swelling, tenderness, and erythema over the involved bone. Fever may be low-grade or absent. Diagnosis can be made by history, physical examination, radiographic studies of the spine, bone scan, blood cultures, erythrocyte sedimentation rate, complete blood count, needle aspiration of the intervertebral disk space, or biopsy of infected bone. *Staphylococcus aureus* is the most common causative organism, but gram-negative bacteria can also cause osteomyelitis (most common after a urinary tract infection).

176. The answer is C. (*Bonica, pp 260, 495.*) Postherpetic neuralgia is pain that persists in a dermatomal pattern long after the vesicular eruptions of an acute herpes zoster infection have healed. Acute herpes zoster is caused by the varicella-zoster virus. On initial infection, the varicella-zoster virus will produce chickenpox. After symptoms subside, the varicella-zoster virus will lie dormant in neural ganglia until physical conditions such as immune compromise or advancing age allow its expression as acute herpes zoster. Herpes simplex types I and II may also produce painful eruptions (cold sores and genital herpes) but are not as severe as zoster and do not follow dermatomal distributions.

177. The answer is B. (*Bonica, pp 1457–1458.*) Waddell described five signs that indicate an increased likelihood that the patient's low back pain is nonorganic. Psychosocial factors are likely to be the major cause of the patient's pain complaints. Waddell's signs are as follows:

1. Superficial nonanatomic tenderness. If the patient's back pain gets worse with pinching or rolling of the skin, this is a positive Waddell's sign.
2. Axial loading by placing one's hand on the patient's head or rotation of the hips and shoulders without twisting the torso. If the patient complains of low back pain in these situations, this is a positive Waddell's sign.
3. Documenting a discrepancy between supine straight-leg raising and the ability to extend the leg fully while sitting.
4. A nonphysiologic pain drawing, or disturbance of sensation in a nondermatomal pattern.
5. Pain behaviors grossly out of proportion to the test stimulus, physical examination, and history.

Patients with three or more Waddell's signs do not usually respond to medical or surgical interventions.

178. The answer is C. (*Wall, pp 718–719.*) This patient presents with symptoms of neurogenic claudication caused by spinal stenosis or spondylosis. Neurogenic claudication is characterized by cramping, numbness, and pain that occur with standing or walking. Peripheral vascular claudication is worse after exercise and is not affected by changes in position.

179. The answer is A. (*Bonica, p 724.*) Hot dog headaches can occur after eating frankfurters or other cured meats that contain nitrites. The headache is often pulsatile, and either bifrontal or bitemporal. Facial flushing may also occur. Treatment consists of avoiding cured meats or products that contain nitrites.

180. The answer is C. (*Bonica, p 724.*) The patient is suffering from Chinese restaurant syndrome, which is thought to be caused by monosodium glutamate (MSG). It is characterized by headache and a sensation of tightness around the head and face. Dizziness, nausea, abdominal cramps, and diarrhea may also occur. Approximately 30 percent of people who eat Chinese food containing MSG will develop symptoms of Chinese restaurant syndrome. The mechanism by which MSG causes the headache and other symptoms is unknown.

181. The answer is D. (*Bonica, p 724.*) Ice cream headache occurs in 25 to 30 percent of the general population, and in up to 90 percent of patients with a history of migraine. Intense pain, most often midfrontal, occurs after ingestion of cold foods. The pain usually lasts less than 1 min. Reflex vasospasm is suspected as the cause of the headache.

182. The answer is D. (*Wall, pp 882–883.*) A dysesthesia is an unpleasant, abnormal sensation, whether spontaneous or evoked. A paresthesia is an abnormal sensation (not primarily unpleasant or painful) that can be spontaneous or evoked. Diminished sensitivity to noxious stimuli is called hypoesthesia. Hyperpathia is a painful syndrome in which there is an increased threshold to perception of a stimulus. However, once the threshold is reached (most frequently by a repetitive stimulus), there is an increased reaction to the stimulus.

183. The answer is E. *(Bonica, p 1300.)* Pain in the left iliac region is frequently caused by acute salpingitis, chronic salpingo-oophoritis, ectopic pregnancy, twisted ovarian cyst, ruptured graafian follicle, acute oophoritis, ulcerative colitis, acute diverticulitis, left lower ureteral calculus, volvulus of the sigmoid, and intestinal obstruction. Meckel's diverticulitis is a common cause of pain in the *right* iliac region.

184. The answer is B. *(Bonica, p 1154.)* Cutting, tearing, or crushing abdominal viscera does not result in pain or in other perceptible sensation. The visceral peritoneum derives its nerve supply from the autonomic nerves supplying the viscera. In conscious patients, pain can be elicited by noxious stimuli applied to the parietal peritoneum, but these stimuli are ineffective when applied to the visceral peritoneum or the viscera themselves. Pain is produced by tension or stretch applied to the viscera or the visceral peritoneum, such as overdistention of the hollow viscera or traction of the mesentery that stretches the nerve plexus in the walls of the organs or the nerves in the mesentery. Other effective stimuli are spasm or contraction of the visceral muscle, ischemia, and inflammation, which lowers the pain threshold of nerve endings.

185. The answer is C. *(Raj, p 116.)* Patrick's maneuver is performed by placing the heel of the painful limb on the knee of the opposite extremity. The thigh is then pressed downward. If pain occurs in the hip (Patrick's sign), this suggests hip joint disease. It is a useful test to help aid in the diagnosis of painful syndromes of the hip, groin, and thigh.

186. The answer is D. *(Wiener, pp 382, 394.)* Spondylolisthesis (slippage) of L5 over S1 occurs in 50 percent of people with a history of spondylolysis. It is usually grade 1 (less than 30 percent). Acute symptoms may develop when the slippage occurs. A standing lateral radiograph of the lumbosacral spine will reveal the degree of slippage. Conservative therapy of bed rest and analgesics may ameliorate symptoms. If disabling symptoms persist, spinal fusion may be necessary.

187–189. The answers are 187-C, 188-A, 189-B. *(Brown, pp 15–21.)* The patient described has triceps weakness associated with a herniated disk at C6–C7. The triceps muscle is innervated by roots of C6, C7, and C8, which come together in the brachial plexus to form the posterior cord. The primary branch of the posterior cord is the radial nerve. Other small terminal branches of the posterior cord include the subscapular, thoracodorsal, and axillary nerves.

190. The answer is D. *(Wiener, p 382.)* The most common site of linear fatigue fracture of the pars interarticularis (spondylolysis) is at L5. Fractures occur less commonly at L2, L3, and L4. Patients complain of lower back and paravertebral pain with associated muscle spasm. Pain often radiates to the buttocks or thighs. Patients are often young and athletic. In children and young adults, pars fractures are treated by body cast or corset immobilization for 6 to 8 weeks. Spondylolisthesis (slippage) of L5 over S1 occurs in 50 percent of patients with spondylolysis.

191. The answer is C. *(Wiener, p 344.)* All the diseases listed are associated with abdominal pain. However, hereditary angioedema is the only one that produces a thumbprinting pattern of the small bowel due to edema. It is a hereditary condition caused by low C4 and C1 esterase inhibitors. Signs and symptoms include abdominal pain due to partial obstruction from edema of the bowel wall; intravascular fluid leakage into tissues, causing an elevation of hematocrit and white blood cell count; nonpitting, brawny angioedema of the face, hands, feet, and trunk; postural hypotension due to third space fluid losses; and possible airway obstruction due to laryngeal edema. Patients can be treated successfully with danazol.

192. The answer is C. *(Wiener, p 145.)* Patients with ankylosing spondylitis may have erosion of the odontoid or destruction of the transverse ligament, which may allow C1 subluxation on C2. Patients will complain of neck, occipital, and shoulder pain. The subluxation is usually mild in these patients. Plain radiographs and MRI should be obtained to confirm the diagnosis. Treatment is symptomatic.

193. The answer is A. (*Wiener, p 12.*) Posttraumatic dysautonomic cephalgia can occur after an injury to the neck. If damage to the sympathetic nerves occurs, patients may complain of a severe, unilateral, aching, and throbbing headache that lasts for hours to days and is associated with mydriasis and hyperhidrosis on the painful side. As the headache resolves, ptosis and miosis occur. The headaches often begin several weeks after the initial injury and may occur as frequently as several times a month. Treatment with beta blockers has been helpful.

194. The answer is B. (*Wiener, p 19.*) Drug-induced aseptic meningitis may be due to a hypersensitivity reaction to drugs such as sulindac, ibuprofen, tolmetin, trimethoprim-sulfamethoxazole, azathioprine, penicillin, isoniazid, phenazopyridine, and sulfonamides. Facial swelling, urticaria, pruritus, and conjunctivitis may also occur along with the fever, headache, vomiting, and depressed level of consciousness. Symptoms usually resolve rapidly after the causative drug is eliminated. CSF studies show predominance of neutrophils and low or normal glucose. Patients with lupus, Sjögren's syndrome, or mixed connective tissue disease have the greatest risk of developing drug-induced meningitis. The incidence is higher in women.

195. The answer is D. (*Wiener, pp 30–31.*) Exertional headache has an incidence greater than 100 per 100,000 persons and is considered a common disease entity. Brain tumor associated with headache is uncommon (5 to 10 per 100,000 persons). Multiple sclerosis and pheochromocytoma are rare diseases, occurring in 4 to 5 per 100,000 persons. Exertional headaches may occur after high-intensity athletic effort, exercise at high altitudes, or low-intensity exercise in persons who are not well conditioned. The headaches vary in intensity, character, and location. They may begin during or immediately after exercise or may occur 1 to 24 h after exercise. The headaches are relatively benign in most cases and may be prevented or treated with NSAIDS. However, up to 10 percent of patients with exertional headache have Chiari malformation or other pathology, which includes subdural hematoma and brain tumor.

196. The answer is B. (*Wiener, p 126.*) Eagle's syndrome, also known as stylohyoid syndrome, may occur after tonsillectomy. Fibrosis occurs around an elongated styloid process, impinges on the carotid sheath, and causes pain in the upper neck, jaw, face, ears, sternocleidomastoid, or temporal region. Pain can be exacerbated by swallowing, talking, or turning the head. Surgical removal of the styloid may be necessary.

197. The answer is D. (*Wiener, p 142.*) Seventy percent of cervical radiculopathies involve C7, 20 percent involve C6, and 10 percent involve C5 or C8. Pain radiation to the forearm and hand are nonspecific. Careful documentation of reflexes, motor weakness, and hypoesthesia or paresthesias will help to identify the involved nerve root(s).

198. The answer is B. (*Wiener, p 142.*) The description is classic for a C5 nerve root lesion. A C4 lesion is not usually associated with arm pain or muscle weakness. A C6 lesion is associated with arm pain, sensory abnormalities, weakness of biceps and branchialis muscles, and abnormal biceps and brachioradialis reflexes. C7 lesions cause arm and hand pain, sensory abnormalities, a decreased or absent triceps reflex, and weakness of the triceps extensor carpi ulnaris and radialis.

199. The answer is C. (*Wiener, p 142.*) The patient presents with symptoms consistent with C7 involvement. C5 nerve root lesions are not usually associated with hand pain or sensory abnormalities. There is deltoid weakness and an abnormal biceps reflex. C6 lesions may cause pain in the entire arm with sensory abnormalities in the thumb and index fingers, biceps and brachialis muscle weakness, and abnormal biceps and brachioradialis reflexes. C8 lesions cause pain in the medial arm and forearm, which may radiate into the ring and little fingers. Patients may complain of sensory abnormalities in the ring and little fingers as well as pain. Reflexes are normal. There is weakness of the intrinsic muscles of the hand.

200. The answer is B. *(Wiener, p 145.)* C6 nerve root lesions often cause weakness of the biceps and brachialis muscles. The biceps reflex is diminished. The brachioradialis reflex is absent or inverted. An inverted brachioradialis reflex describes the condition in which the fingers flex but the elbow fails to flex. Patients may complain of numbness and tingling in the thumb and index finger. Pain perception may involve the entire arm.

201. The answer is D. *(Wiener, p 142.)* In addition to the symptoms described, C8 nerve root lesions may also cause numbness and tingling in the ring and little fingers. C5 lesions do not cause hand pain or sensory abnormalities, but they do cause deltoid weakness and an abnormal biceps reflex. C6 lesions are associated with sensory abnormalities of the thumb and index finger, weakness of the biceps and brachialis muscles, and abnormal biceps and brachioradialis reflexes. C7 lesions are associated with numbness and tingling in the index and middle fingers, weakness of the extensors, and an abnormal triceps reflex.

202. The answer is A. *(Wiener, p 142.)* All the organisms listed have been known to cause epidural abscess. However, *Staphylococcus aureus* is by far the most common. Cases of *Pseudomonas*-infected epidural abscess have been described in intravenous drug abusers. Epidural abscess caused by gram-negative rods has arisen in patients with documented urinary tract infections. Streptococcal species have also been found to cause epidural abscess in rare cases.

203. The answer is C. *(Wiener, p 146.)* Botulinum toxin A (Botox) may be a useful treatment in some cases of torticollis. Torticollis is caused by spasm of the sternocleidomastoid muscles. Lateral pharyngeal or retropharyngeal space infections, cervical lymphadenitis, and pyogenic or tuberculous osteomyelitis of the cervical spine are infectious processes that may be associated with torticollis. Acute myositis, which can occur after excessive muscular use, viral illness, and sleeping in a draft or with the neck cramped, can also cause torticollis. Accessory nerve neuritis, herniated cervical disk, syringomyelia, cerebellar tonsillar herniation, facet joint disease, vertebral fractures or subluxations, phenothiazine ingestion, and hyperthyroidism have all been cited as causes of torticollis.

204. The answer is C. *(Wiener, p 147.)* The patient is suffering from occipital neuralgia, which probably occurred as a result of a whiplash injury sustained at the time of his motor vehicle accident in which there was injury to the ganglion and root of C2. Other causes of occipital neuralgia are a compressive blow over the occipital nerve, degenerative arthritis of the atlantoaxial joint, entrapment of the greater occipital nerve by lymphadenopathy or vascular anomaly, and occupations involving neck hyperextension and rotation.

205. The answer is D. *(Bonica, p 631. Raj, pp 280–281.)* The patient's symptoms are most consistent with carpal tunnel syndrome, which is due to entrapment of the median nerve at the wrist. Prolongation of distal motor latency may be seen on EMG. It primarily affects women, who may complain of a pricking numbness of the fingers and hands. Pregnant women and patients with systemic diseases that cause tissue swelling, such as endocrine disorders or collagen vascular diseases, are at increased risk of developing carpal tunnel syndrome.

206. The answer is C. *(Wall, p 796.)* Patients may complain of diffuse pain and tenderness of muscles and joints following a reduction in the dose of corticosteroid. The symptoms may occur during a rapid or slow taper in patients who have been on steroids for even a short period of time. It is postulated that steroid withdrawal may sensitize nociceptors and mechanoreceptors by an unknown mechanism.

207. The answer is B. *(Wall, p 713.)* The geniculate ganglion is located in the roof of the temporal bone. The nervus intermedius, which is a branch of cranial nerve VII, has its cell bodies in the geniculate ganglion. It supplies sensory afferents to the tympanic membrane, external auditory canal, skin in the area between the ear and mastoid process, and some deep structures of the head and neck. Young to middle-aged adults are most commonly affected. It is less common than glossopharyngeal neuralgia. Ramsay Hunt syndrome is geniculate neuralgia associated with the occurrence of a herpes zoster–type vesicular rash in the external ear and around the mastoid area, often accompanied by ipsilateral facial paralysis.

208. The answer is D. (*Wall, p 892.*) Approximately 1 to 2 percent of stroke patients develop central pain. It is frequently characterized as burning, aching, and pricking. Neurologic signs such as sensory abnormalities, paresis, and ataxia are present in the majority of patients with central poststroke syndrome.

209. The answer is B. (*Wall, pp 896–897.*) Syringomyelia is a rare disease with a very high incidence of central pain (73 percent). The patients may complain of pain in one of the upper extremities or occasionally both extremities. Thoracic pain may be reported. Pain in the lower extremities has also been documented in a few patients with syringomyelia. The pain is described as burning, aching, or pressing in nature. Sensory abnormalities are found on examination (i.e., abnormal temperature, touch, and vibration senses and kinesthesia). Treatment consists of drugs and therapies used to treat central pain due to other disease processes. TENS may be helpful, but dorsal column stimulation has not been shown to be effective.

210. The answer is B. (*Wall, p 798.*) AHZ occurs more frequently in patients with hematologic or lymphoproliferative cancers, and in those patients who receive immunosuppressive therapies. The location of the cancer is associated with the site of AHZ occurrence. Patients with breast or lung cancer are more likely to develop thoracic AHZ, those with head and neck cancer tend to develop facial AHZ, and those with gynecologic or urologic tumors frequently develop lumbar or sacral AHZ. AHZ also occurs most often in areas that have been previously irradiated.

211. The answer is C. (*Wall, p 700.*) The patient is suffering from trigeminal neuralgia (tic douloureux). Atypical facial pain is characterized by a constant, burning or aching pain. Postherpetic neuralgia is usually preceded by acute herpes zoster lesions on the face and is a constant, burning, often lancinating pain. Vascular pain can be intermittent; it is usually throbbing or burning in nature and is not usually associated with a nonpainful trigger stimulus as is trigeminal neuralgia.

212. The answer is A. (*Wall, pp 671–673.*) Chronic renal failure is associated with large myelinated fiber loss, which is rarely painful. Small myelinated and unmyelinated fiber loss is found in diabetic neuropathy, Fabry's disease, amyloid neuropathy, and hereditary sensory neuropathy. Patients with these disorders may complain of a burning, aching, lancinating pain.

213. The answer is A. (*Wall, p 620.*) Diabetic neuropathy is associated with loss of small fibers. Isoniazid neuropathy, pellagra neuropathy, and hypothyroid neuropathy are all painful polyneuropathies associated with the selective loss of neural fibers of large diameter. Isoniazid may cause distal numbness and tingling followed by a deep ache or burning pain as the myelinated fibers are selectively damaged. Lower extremity sensorimotor neuropathy and cutaneous hyperesthesia may also be present. Pellagra neuropathy is due to niacin deficiency. Sensorimotor neuropathy of the lower extremities with painful feet, tender calf muscles, and cutaneous hyperesthesia occurs. Hypothyroid sensorimotor neuropathy is associated with painful feet and paresthesias of the hands.

214. The answer is B. (*Wall, p 669.*) Congenital analgesia is a syndrome in which impairment of pain sensation predisposes to tissue-damaging injury. Patients often present with damage to the tongue and hands. Pain and thermal perception are impaired. Other sensory modalities are not affected. The children also do not sweat, and this may lead to episodes of elevated body temperature. There is also a high incidence of subnormal intelligence. The pathology noted on autopsy reveals total absence of small dorsal root ganglion cells and small fibers in the dorsal roots and Lissauer's tract.

215–216. The answers are 215-D, 216-D. (*Wall, pp 725–728, 731–732. Raj, pp 305–306.*) Arachnoiditis may develop in patients with chronic lumbosacral root compression due to disk protrusion or spinal stenosis; after bacterial, viral, or fungal meningitis; after hemorrhage due to trauma, vascular malformation, lumbar puncture, or spinal surgery; and after intrathecal injection of irritant chemicals, such as iophendylate

(Pantopaque), steroid (methylprednisolone with polyethylene glycol), and possibly local anesthetics with methylparaben (a preservative). Nerve roots may be encased in dense, fibrous adhesions within the canal. Radicular pain is not uncommon and may involve more than one nerve root.

Treatment is very discouraging. Epidural steroids provide transient relief. Surgical or chemical lysis of intradural adhesions may also provide some degree of relief. Conservative treatment consisting of NSAIDs, tricyclic antidepressants (TCAs) for burning pain, and anticonvulsants for lancinating pain due to neuropathy secondary to chronic nerve compression may provide some relief. Narcotics have been used by some practitioners with some success. Spinal cord stimulation has been effective long term in approximately 50 percent of patients with arachnoiditis.

217. **The answer is A.** (*Tollison, p 260.*) Posttraumatic headaches can occur in patients who have had even mild head trauma or flexion-extension injuries. The headaches may be throbbing or nonthrobbing, intermittent or continuous, and are usually unilateral and often occipitocervical. Occasionally, they will present as intermittent, unilateral neck or orbital pain and may be confused with cluster headaches. Nonheadache symptoms may include vertigo, depression and anxiety, impaired memory and attention span, insomnia, and decreased motivation. Treatment consists of counseling, biofeedback, physical therapy, TENS, tricyclic antidepressants, beta blockers or calcium-channel blockers, and NSAIDs. Intermittent, acute headaches may be treated like acute migraine. Focal tenderness of neck muscles may respond to injections of local anesthetics and steroids. Neuralgic symptoms may be treated with anticonvulsants or baclofen. Surgical decompression or neurectomy has been successful in some patients.

218. **The answer is D.** (*Bonica, p 722.*) The prevalence of giant cell arteritis (temporal arteritis) increases after age 50 and occurs twice as often in women. Patients complain of temporal headache of a constant, boring quality, which may be relieved with aspirin. They may also have symmetric arthralgias and myalgias, general malaise, anorexia, low-grade fever, claudication of jaw muscles, and visual loss due to ischemia of the optic nerve and retina. Facial and temporal artery pulsations may be absent. Blindness and stroke have occurred. The diagnosis is confirmed by temporal artery biopsy. Patients with giant cell arteritis also have an increased ESR. Treatment is with corticosteroids. In the presence of intolerable side effects, azathioprine has been used with some success. Patients should be on the lowest dose of medication that will suppress the ESR, which should be checked regularly. Rise in the ESR may indicate potential relapse.

219. **The answer is D.** (*Raj, p 579.*) Primary causes of coccygeal pain include sprained ligaments, dislocation fracture, childbirth, osteoarthritis of the coccygeal joints, and subluxation of the coccyx. Metastases and external compression by a tumor mass represent 2 percent of cases. Referred pain may occur in patients with lumbar disk disease, cauda equina syndrome, arachnoiditis, spinal cord tumor, perirectal abscess or fistula, pilonidal cyst, pelvic inflammatory disease or tumor, vaginismus, levator syndrome, and psychoneurosis.

220. **The answer is E.** (*Tollison, pp 440–441.*) The patient has meralgia paresthetica, entrapment of the lateral femoral cutaneous nerve of the thigh. The nerve is derived from the L2 and L3 roots. It penetrates the psoas muscle and traverses the pelvis to the anterosuperior iliac spine, where it exits beneath the inguinal ligament. Meralgia paresthetica is most frequent in conditions in which the abdomen protrudes over the anterosuperior iliac spine, such as pregnancy, obesity, and liver disease. Direct trauma to the nerve, tight jeans, or standing at attention may also cause meralgia paresthetica by direct pressure or stretch of the lateral femoral cutaneous nerve. Patients may complain of burning, itching, feelings of cold, numbness, or hyperesthesias of the anterolateral thigh. Most patients recover spontaneously over weeks to months. Elimination of the cause (such as weight loss, wearing loose clothing, delivery of the baby) will usually provide symptomatic relief. Local anesthetic may be of benefit in confirming the diagnosis and in decreasing the pain. Sectioning of the nerve is not recommended, for this may lead to the development of painful neuromas.

221. **The answer is D.** (*Tollison, pp 246, 247, 249.*) The pain pathways for structures in the anterior and middle fossae follow the ipsilateral trigeminal nerve, usually referred to the frontal, temporal, or parietal region.

The posterior fossa is innervated by the ipsilateral cervical nerves I, II, and III, as well as the glossopharyngeal and vagus nerves. Pain from posterior fossa structures is usually felt in the occipital region. The symptoms listed are classic for posterior fossa tumor.

Cluster headaches are more common in males and are always unilateral and usually periorbital. Attacks last 10 min to 3 h, occur one to six times per day, and are characterized as very severe pain.

Migraine headaches are more common in females and usually, but not always, unilateral. Attacks that cause the patient to move about restlessly occur one to eight times per month and last 4 to 48 h. Migraines may be associated with prodromal symptoms, such as visual disturbances or food cravings. The patient may complain of nausea and vomiting and have photophobia. Lying still may help control the pain.

Tolosa-Hunt syndrome is an intense, sharp, or aching ocular pain. It may be associated with arteritis or granulomatous lesions within the orbit. The pain may be followed by several days of ophthalmoplegia and diplopia.

222–223. The answers are 222-D, 223-C. (*Bonica, pp 1273–1274.*) Acute intermittent porphyria is due to an autosomal dominant enzyme defect that results in decreased uroporphyrinogen synthetase. Acute attacks of mental or abdominal neurologic symptoms can be precipitated by drugs, starvation, infection, or sex hormones. Symptoms of nervous system damage rarely occur before puberty. Acute attacks may last from days to months and vary in intensity. Diagnosis is made by urinary analysis for excess porphobilinogen. Urine chromatography or the Watson-Schwartz or Hoesch tests can be performed to confirm the diagnosis. In the clinical setting, the easiest test is to obtain a urine sample and expose it to light and air, which will cause the initially colorless porphobilinogen to break down to porphobilin, which is dark brown in color. Treatment consists of avoiding the precipitating factors listed above. If patients must undergo surgery, sodium pentothal and other barbiturates should be avoided. During an attack, patients suffering from severe pain may be managed with IV PCA narcotic analgesics, phenothiazines, or epidural analgesia to control symptoms.

224. The answer is C. (*Bonica, p 1407.*) The loads on an L3 disk in a 70-kg person are as follows: supine 30 kg; standing 70 kg; upright sitting without support 100 kg; walking 85 kg; bending sideways 95 kg; jumping 110 kg; bending forward 20° 120 kg; lifting 20 kg with back straight and knees bent 210 kg; lifting 20 kg with back bent and knees straight 340 kg.

225. The answer is D. (*Bonica, p 1407.*) Maximum load on the disk occurs when a person is sitting against a 90° back rest without lumbar support. There is slightly less load on the lumbar spine when one sits at 90° with lumbar support. There is even less load on the lumbar spine when the back of the chair is inclined to 110° without lumbar support. There is least pressure on the lumbar spine with the back of the chair at 100° with a lumbar support.

226. The answer is A. (*Bonica, pp 1271–1272.*) Sickle cell disease is a chronic hemolytic anemia. It occurs primarily in the black population because of genetic transmission of a molecular lesion of hemoglobin; 0.15 percent of black children are homozygous for this trait and manifest symptoms of sickle cell disease. Valine is substituted for glutamic acid at the sixth position in the beta chain of hemoglobin. The sickle hemoglobin is fragile and thereby less able to withstand the trauma of circulation, infection, and dehydration. Patients with sickle cell disease suffer from recurrent, painful vaso-occlusive attacks, which may result in progressive infarction of the liver, spleen, gallbladder, and lungs. Complications associated with these crises lead to shorter life expectancy. Diagnosis of the disease is made by history, physical examination, and blood electrophoresis. Homozygotes have almost all HbS with a variable amount of HbF (fetal hemoglobin). They have no HbA. Heterozygotes, patients with sickle cell trait, have more HbA than HbS, and as such will not experience hemolysis, painful crises, and thrombotic complications associated with sickle cell disease. Therapy consists of symptomatic treatment. Splenectomy and hematinics are not helpful.

227. The answer is D. (*Bonica, pp 874–876.*) Thoracic outlet syndrome may be due to a cervical rib, abnormal first thoracic rib, hypertrophy of the scalenus anterior, abnormal insertion of the scalenus medius, bands in Sibson's fascia, or costoclavicular abnormalities. There is usually involvement of the subclavian vessels and brachial plexus (most commonly C8–T1). The degree of vascular and neurologic dysfunction is variable.

Patients may complain of radicular pain or a poorly localized, deep, aching pain under the arm. Cold weather, lifting heavy objects, working with arms over the head, and repetitive movements may worsen symptoms. Pain may occur for years before any neurologic symptoms or signs develop. Diagnosis is made by physical examination and radiologic studies of the neck and chest. Treatment is conservative if there is no significant vascular or neurologic compromise.

228. **The answer is C.** (*Bonica, p 679.*) Tic douloureux, or classic trigeminal neuralgia, occurs most commonly in the V2 division (44 percent), then the V3 division (36 percent), and least often in the V1 division (20 percent). Tic pain often occurs in more than one division of the trigeminal nerve. The most common combination is V2 and V3 and the least common is V1 and V3. The trigger area is always on the same side of the pain and is usually in the sensory distribution of the trigeminal nerve. It may actually be outside of the trigeminal division or divisions where the pain occurs. For example, touching a trigger in the V1 division may precipitate pain in the V2 trigeminal dermatome.

229. **The answer is D.** (*Raj, p 410.*) The stress response is a complex hormonal and neurologic sequence mediated via adrenergic sympathetic pathways. Elevated sympathetic efferent activity—along with elevated serum epinephrine, norepinephrine, growth hormone, cortisol, renin, aldosterone, and antidiuretic hormone levels—leads to tachycardia, hypertension, and increased muscle blood flow. The predominance of catabolic response leads to hyperglycemia secondary to increased glycogenolysis, lipolysis, and proteolysis in the face of decreased glucose turnover.

230. **The answer is D.** (*Bonica, pp 407, 1098–1100.*) Radiation-induced fibrosis of the connective tissue surrounding the brachial plexus can cause compression and ischemic neuropathy. Symptoms have developed 6 months to 20 years after radiation therapy. The patient complains of deafferentation-type pain. It is characterized as progressively increasing, diffuse, and burning. Other symptoms and signs may include numbness, paresthesias, dysesthesias, and C5–C6 motor weakness. There are significant differences in symptoms in patients with metastatic plexopathy versus radiation plexopathy. Most patients with metastatic plexopathy develop sensory changes in C8–T1 distribution versus C5–C6 in radiation plexopathy. Patients with metastatic plexopathy also have a much higher incidence of Horner's syndrome, lymphedema and swelling of the painful limb, and development of epidural deposits.

231. **The answer is D.** (*Tollison, pp 385–387.*) Scrotal pain or pain in the inguinal area is often associated with pathology of the testicle or epididymis. A careful history and physical examination should be performed to rule out acute conditions such as testicular torsion, infection of the epididymis or testicle, and fracture of a portion of the testicle after trauma. Testicular cancer is most common in men 20 to 40 years of age. Urinalysis will provide information regarding inflammatory or infectious causes of pain. If examination of the testicle reveals that it is elevated in the scrotum close to the external inguinal ring, torsion exists and may be a surgical emergency. If a portion of the testicle has been fractured in a traumatic event, the painful necrotic portion of the testicle may require excision and anastomosis of the tunica albuginea to preserve function of the remaining portion of the testicle. Early testicular cancer is usually nonpainful, but it is frequently associated with epididymitis. After appropriate treatment of the infection/inflammation, ultrasound and possibly a testicular biopsy should be performed to rule out testicular cancer. Paraphimosis is a condition in which the retracted foreskin forms a constricting band at the base of the glans. This may be associated with penile pain.

232. **The answer is B.** (*Tollison, pp 385–386.*) In testicular torsion, the urinalysis will be normal and there is usually no elevation in temperature. Radioactive testicular scans will reveal decreased blood supply to the testicle, which is diagnostic of testicular torsion and is considered a surgical emergency if the torsion cannot be untwisted within the scrotal sac. A testicular ultrasound also may be helpful in the evaluation of the scrotal structures. Testicular biopsy is usually done to evaluate masses that are either palpated or revealed on ultrasound and to rule out testicular cancer. Traumatic injury to the testicle can be treated with ice, elevation, and immobilization. Needle aspiration of a hydrocele can be done but is not recommended.

TYPES OF PAIN ANSWERS

233. The answer is D. (*Bonica, pp 1628–1629.*) Patients with successfully treated reflex sympathetic dystrophy should minimize trauma to the affected part and be careful not to reinjure themselves. They are at increased risk of developing reflex sympathetic dystrophy in the previously affected limb and, in some cases, in other parts of the body as well. Normal activity is essential to maintain bone mass and function. Properly fitting shoes that are supportive and nonbinding should be worn. Reevaluation and treatment should be reinstituted as soon as possible if symptoms return.

234. The answer is B. (*Bonica, p 1469.*) Pain from spinal stenosis is caused by narrowing of the spinal canal due to degenerative changes in the joints and disks. This often results in multidermatomal leg pain in one or both legs, buttocks, and low back. Movements that open the spinal canal, such as leaning forward (walking uphill, riding a bicycle), will often decrease the pain. Movements that decrease the size of the spinal canal, such as walking downhill, will increase the pain.

235. The answer is D. (*Tollison, p 450.*) In one study, most patients with clinical signs and symptoms of reflex sympathetic dystrophy had positive delayed image bone scans (22 of 23 patients). Positive blood pool angiograms were also found in 12 of 23; 10 of 23 had positive radionuclide angiograms. Almost half of the patients had positive early phase bone scans.

236. The answer is B. (*Tollison, p 32.*) Median nerve entrapment at the wrist is called carpal tunnel syndrome. However, electrodiagnostic evaluation (electromyography and nerve conduction studies) should be performed to rule out median nerve entrapment at the elbow and entrapment of the radial nerve, ulnar nerve, or both. Patients with carpal tunnel syndrome usually present with paresthesias of the hand; they occasionally also complain of shoulder pain, hand weakness, and the tendency to drop small objects. The symptoms may awaken the patient at night and be most severe upon arising in the morning.

237. The answer is D. (*Raj, p 551.*) At least 30 percent of patients with AIDS will suffer from a painful, predominantly sensory neuropathy, which is believed to be due to direct viral HIV infection. A progressive axonal degeneration and demyelination occurs. Patients frequently complain of painful soles of the feet, paresthesias, or sensations of cold or burning pain.

238. The answer is C (2,4). (*Bonica, p 782.*) Eagle's syndrome, also known as stylohyoid syndrome, is caused by dystrophic calcification of the stylohyoid ligament. Pain occurs during mandibular movement or with twisting of the neck. There are no trigger points, and pain is absent when the mouth is closed. The pain is stabbing, with radiation from the tonsil area to the temporomandibular joint and base of the tongue. Treatment consists of surgical excision of the stylohyoid ligament and the elongated styloid or cervical process, if present.

239. The answer is A (1,2,3). (*Wall, p 717.*) S1 nerve root injury may be associated with weakness of plantar flexion, occasional cramping in the calf, and absent ankle jerk. Atrophy of the gastrocnemius, soleus, and hamstrings may occur. Sagging of the gluteal fold and loss of gluteal muscle tone also suggest S1 involvement. Radicular pain in the knee is suggestive of L3 injury.

240. The answer is A (1,2,3). (*Raj, p 74.*) Useful therapeutic modalities in the treatment of pain from terminal disease include anti-inflammatory agents, narcotics, anxiolytics, antidepressants, and neural blockade. Also essential to treating terminal pain are psychological support, family support, and a multidisciplinary approach to managing this complex problem.

241. The answer is A (1,2,3). (*Raj, p 75.*) Chronic pain is not biologically useful. It has poorly defined peripheral nociceptive mechanisms and peripheral neural transmission and poorly defined central connections and central pathways. The acute physiologic stress response is not present.

242. **The answer is A (1,2,3).** (*Raj, p 877.*) Patients experiencing deafferentation pain commonly complain of numbness, burning (causalgia, caustic pain), coldness, or, in severe cases, crushing, tearing, or ripping sensations. Their pain is usually constant, unremitting, and accompanied by prominent suffering. Narcotic analgesics characteristically do not afford much relief beyond their sedative and mood-altering effects. Also, further destruction of neural tissue via neurosurgical intervention rarely gives the patient lasting relief and may result in an even more widespread deafferentation pain state.

243. **The answer is A (1,2,3).** (*Wall, pp 991–995.*) Peripheral neuropathies, regardless of their cause, have several characteristic signs and symptoms: paresthesias and dysesthesias, sensory loss, loss or diminution of tendon reflexes, and impaired motor function. Not all peripheral neuropathies are painful, and when pain is associated with a peripheral neuropathy, it usually is not a distinguishing feature of the neuropathy.

244. **The answer is C (2,4).** (*Raj, p 74.*) Terminal pain, a variant of acute pain, is biologically harmful and usually involves well-defined tissue damage. Other types of pain related to therapy can coexist. The stress response is harmful.

245. **The answer is B (1,3).** (*Bonica, pp 1457–1458.*) Waddell's signs are five types of findings that greatly increase the likelihood that psychosocial factors are playing a major role in the patient's complaints. The five findings include superficial, nonanatomic tenderness; a positive simulation response; a discrepancy between results of examination of the same body part in two different positions; nonphysiologic regional disturbances of sensation, pain, or weakness; and a positive test for overreaction. Patients with three or more positive test results do not respond favorably to any form of physical treatment, and surgery is not often beneficial.

246. **The answer is B (1,3).** (*Wall, p 507.*) Attacks of CPH resemble those of cluster headache. However, they last for a shorter time, are more frequent, have no nocturnal preponderance, occur mostly in females, and are responsive to indomethacin. The average attack lasts 15 min, and as many as 40 per 24 h may occur.

247. **The answer is E (all).** (*Raj, pp 547–550.*) Neurologic disease can be either a direct result of HIV infection or a direct or indirect result of HIV immunosuppression. Early clinical manifestations of HIV encephalopathy include cognitive symptoms, behavioral changes, and motor symptoms. Late manifestations include frank dementia, seizures, and pyramidal tract signs. Painful syndromes in patients with AIDS that involve the peripheral nervous system include Guillain-Barré syndrome, postherpetic neuralgia, and a predominant sensory neuropathy.

248. **The answer is A (1,2,3).** (*Cousins, p 80.*) Plasma concentrations of alpha-1-acid glycoprotein have been found to be considerably elevated in patients with cancer, chronic pain, trauma, and uremia. They are also elevated in patients receiving renal transplants and in postoperative and postmyocardial infarction patients. The low plasma concentrations of alpha-1-acid glycoprotein in neonates are associated with much lower binding of local anesthetic compared with that in adult plasma.

249. **The answer is B (1,3).** (*Wall, pp 669, 672–674.*) Patients suffering from myeloma may complain of a painful sensorimotor neuropathy. Loss of myelinated fibers of all sizes and of unmyelinated fibers occurs. Alcoholic neuropathy is also associated with loss of all sizes of nerve fibers. Patients may complain of a burning pain; tenderness in the legs and feet is more common than upper extremity symptoms. Fabry's disease is a rare lipid storage disorder in which there is selective loss of small nerve fibers. A painful peripheral neuropathy may be the presenting feature. Tangier disease is a rare, familial alpha-lipoprotein deficiency associated with selective loss of pain sensation.

250. **The answer is E (all).** (*Wall, p 745.*) Typical findings in T1 root (i.e., T1–T2 disk) compression include pain in the neck, medial scapula, and anterior chest; subjective numbness in the ulnar aspect of the forearm; weakness of the intrinsic muscles of the hand; and normal deep tendon reflexes. Occasionally, Horner's syndrome (miosis, anhidrosis, and ptosis) can be caused by compression of the sympathetic nerves.

251. The answer is E (all). (*Raj, p 73.*) Certain alterations of neurologic structure and function may result in pain. Metabolic changes of diabetes or mercury poisoning may produce a painful peripheral neuropathy. Viral damage (herpes zoster, late poliomyelitis, and Guillain-Barré syndrome) may also produce painful states. Trauma to peripheral nerves can lead to neuropathic pain from neuromas, causalgia, or phantom pain.

252. The answer is B (1,3). (*Raj, pp 74–75.*) Clinical examples of neuropathic pain syndromes include tic douloureux, phantom limb pain, postherpetic neuralgia, thalamic syndrome, nerve root avulsion, and causalgia. Dyspareunia and vaginismus are classified as psychogenic pain disorders in the third edition of the *Diagnostic and Statistical Manual of Mental Disorders (DSM-III)*.

253. The answer is A (1,2,3). (*Raj, p 414.*) Ketamine produces a profound analgesia and may be used in high doses as the sole agent for emergency and trauma surgery. At lower doses it can be used as an analgesic. This agent possesses sympathomimetic action, which may be beneficial in injured patients with a depressed cardiovascular system because of shock. Ketamine increases intracranial pressure, however, and is contraindicated in head injuries.

254. The answer is C (2,4). (*Cousins, p 340.*) Important diagnostic features of an epidural abscess include severe back pain, local back tenderness, fever, leukocytosis, and an abnormal myelogram with obstruction to flow of contrast medium. Because *Staphylococcus aureus* is the most common infecting organism, antibiotic administration should include treatment for a staphylococcal infection if positive cultures are not available.

255. The answer is A (1,2,3). (*Wall, p 713.*) Glossopharyngeal neuralgia is characterized by paroxysms of lancinating pain in the tonsillar region, base of the tongue, ear and ipsilateral face, neck, or scalp. Patients are almost always older than 20. Attacks may last minutes or seconds and rarely occur at night. The etiology is unknown. Attacks can be triggered by swallowing or by touching the ear, face, or neck. Patients may complain of a constant burning or dull ache between attacks of lancinating pain. Other symptoms that may occur during attacks are cardiac arrhythmias (including arrest), hiccups, seizures, coughing, stridor, and excessive salivation. There is no association between the incidence of tic douloureux and glossopharyngeal neuralgia.

256. The answer is C (2,4). (*Wall, pp 895–896.*) Many SCI patients have chronic pain (42 to 77 percent), which is primarily central. SCI patients also have a high incidence of visceral pain. Treatment is difficult. It usually consists of antiepileptic and antidepressant drugs. TENS may be tried if there is some remaining dorsal column function. Dorsal column stimulation has not been effective. DREZ lesions have been tried with varying success.

257. The answer is A (1,2,3). (*Wall, p 899.*) In a study by Snider and colleagues, 43 out of 105 patients with Parkinson's disease complained of pain, tingling, and numbness. The pain is characterized as intermittent, cramplike, or aching and is not affected by movement or pressure. It is often proximal and most severe in the weakest limb. The pain is related to fluctuations in motor symptoms. If antiparkinsonian medication is adjusted to improve motor symptoms, the pain symptoms also improve. Droperidol is antidopaminergic and can worsen the symptoms of Parkinson's disease.

258. The answer is A (1,2,3). (*Raj, p 207. Tollison, p 246. Wall, p 510.*) Ninety percent of patients with cluster headaches are male. Sixty-five to seventy percent of migraineurs are female. Giant cell arteritis (also called temporal arteritis) is twice as common in females and shows a marked increase in incidence after age 50. In tension headaches, both sexes are affected, but females predominate.

259. The answer is B (1,3). (*Raj, p 505.*) Phantom limb sensation is an almost universal occurrence at some time during the first month following surgery. It is strongest in above-elbow amputations, weakest in below-knee amputations, and more frequent in the dominant limb of double amputees. The incidence of phantom limb sensation increases with the age of the amputee.

260. The answer is E (all). (*Tollison, pp 385–386.*) After a careful history and physical examination is performed, a urinalysis will be helpful in evaluating the patient for inflammatory or infectious processes. Radioactive testicular scans will show decreased blood flow to the testicle in patients with torsion. Testicular ultrasound will reveal masses, and biopsy may be necessary to rule out testicular cancer.

261. The answer is A (1,2,3). (*Tollison, p 387.*) Pain referred to the penile shaft may be due to neuralgias of the ilioinguinal, iliohypogastric, or genitofemoral nerves. Such neuralgias occur most frequently after trauma or surgery. Lateral femoral cutaneous neuralgia (meralgia paresthetica) usually causes pain in the lateral thigh without radiation to the penile shaft. It is also important to remember that referred pain may be felt in the penis from the kidney, ureter, bladder, or prostate.

262. The answer is A (1,2,3). (*Bonica, pp 341–342.*) Reiter's syndrome consists of an asymmetric arthropathy and urethritis or cervicitis, dysentery, mucocutaneous lesions, and inflammatory eye disease. HLA-B27 is present in 80 percent of patients. Treatment consists of NSAIDS, azathioprine, methotrexate, and physical therapy. Antibiotics have not been helpful, though onset of the syndrome may be precipitated by bacterial infections. Plasmapheresis is not used in the treatment of Reiter's syndrome.

263. The answer is E (all). (*Tollison, pp 425–427.*) The causes of painful peripheral neuropathy include AIDS, Sjögren's syndrome, Guillain-Barré syndrome, insulinoma, diabetes, malnutrition, and amyloidosis. It is also caused by ingestion of arsenic, thallium, metronidazole, and nitrofurantoin, and by uremia, ischemia, dysproteinemias, cancer, porphyria, Fabry's disease, and mononeuropathies. The cornerstone of treatment is therapy that eliminates or improves the condition causing the painful neuropathy. The administration of aspirin, acetaminophen, and NSAIDS and the occasional use of narcotics will help to relieve the pain in cases where the neuropathy is transient and will improve once the inciting agent is eliminated or the disease process treated. In cases where neuropathies may be long-standing (e.g., diabetes, AIDS, cancer), medications such as anticonvulsants, tricyclic antidepressants, phenothiazines, calcium-channel blockers, and antiarrhythmics may be helpful.

264. The answer is E (all). (*Tollison, p 387.*) Priapism is a prolonged, painful penile erection that is seen most commonly in patients with chronic diseases such as leukemia and sickle cell disease. It is considered an emergency condition that may result in scarring and erectile impotence if left untreated.

265. The answer is A (1,2,3). (*Tollison, pp 449–451.*) In patients with clinical signs of reflex sympathetic dystrophy, over 80 percent will have positive delayed image bone scans. In some cases, osteoporosis may be seen on plain films, though this finding is not as common as the bone scan results. Response to lumbar sympathetic blockade can be diagnostic as well as therapeutic. Intravenous lidocaine has been used to help guide medication selection and as therapy in patients with neuropathic pain.

266. The answer is A (1,2,3). (*Tollison, p 349.*) Criteria for the diagnosis of acute lumbar radicular syndrome include (1) leg pain (including buttock) as the dominant complaint when compared with back pain; (2) neurologic symptoms in a specific dermatomal distribution; (3) significant straight-leg raising (SLR) findings (SLR less than 50 percent of normal, bowstring discomfort, or crossover pain); and (4) neurologic signs that correspond to specific nerve roots. Evidence of pathology on MRI supports the diagnosis, but is not necessary to make the diagnosis of acute lumbar radicular syndrome. At least two and more often three of the four criteria are present to make the diagnosis of acute lumbar radicular syndrome.

267. The answer is B (1,3). (*Tollison, p 280.*) Raeder's syndrome (paratrigeminal neuralgia) is characterized by frontotemporal pain and oculosympathetic paresis manifest as an incomplete Horner's syndrome. The patient may complain of a migrainous headache that is episodic and lasts hours or days or of a more persistent headache. If the headache is persistent, the patient should be carefully evaluated for the presence of an aneurysm or tumor in the region of the middle fossa or cavernous sinus.

268. The answer is E (all). (*Tollison, p 280.*) Occipital neuralgia is a common cranial neuralgia that may be due to trauma, such as whiplash injuries, entrapment of the C2 nerve root or dorsal root ganglion by paravertebral ligamentous structures, cluster headaches, tumor in the posterior fossa, high cervical spine foramen magnum, herniated cervical intervertebral disk, or metastatic neoplasm at the base of the skull. The pain is usually described as deep, stabbing, and aching in the distribution of C2. It may radiate to the fronto-orbital areas, face, or vertex. Treatment depends on the cause of the occipital neuralgia.

269. The answer is A (1,2,3). (*Tollison, p 281.*) Temporomandibular pain and dysfunction syndrome is characterized by a triad of signs and symptoms: pain and tenderness of the masticatory muscles, joint sounds with jaw opening, and limited mandibular movement. Other signs and symptoms that may be present but are not necessary for diagnosis include bruxism, teeth clenching, ear pain, headache, tinnitus, and dizziness. Conservative, noninvasive treatment with biofeedback, stress management, antidepressants, antianxiety agents, muscle relaxants, NSAIDS, splints, TENS, acupuncture, and trigger point injections is recommended.

270. The answer is E (all). (*Tollison, p 432.*) Carpal tunnel syndrome, entrapment of the median nerve at the wrist, occurs more frequently in pregnant patients; patients with rheumatoid arthritis, gout, amyloidosis, hypothyroidism, hyperthyroidism, and acromegaly; and in patients with vascular shunts placed for hemodialysis. Treatment by conservative measures is usually successful in those patients who have only subjective sensory symptoms or reversible systemic conditions, such as pregnancy or myxedema. Wrist splinting and occasional local injection of steroids may be all that is required. Most other patients will undergo surgical section of the flexor retinaculum to "release" the carpal tunnel.

Pain Assessment

DIRECTIONS: Each question below contains suggested responses. Select the **one best** response.

271. One part of the McGill Pain Questionnaire (MPQ) asks the patient to describe what the pain feels like. Several descriptors are grouped together to characterize the pain. Which of the following would be found in the same category as the term *flickering*?

    (A) Pinching, pressing, gnawing
    (B) Sharp, cutting, lacerating
    (C) Throbbing, beating, pounding
    (D) Jumping, flashing, shooting

272. The Visual Analogue Scale (VAS) consists of a 10-cm line that is labeled "No pain at all" on the left and "The worst pain imaginable" on the right. Patients are asked to mark on the line how strong their pain is at the moment. How is the line divided, if at all?

    (A) 1-cm divisions
    (B) 1-mm divisions
    (C) Divisions numbered 1 through 10
    (D) Divisions numbered 1 through 100
    (E) No divisions

273. All the following are true of the McGill Pain Questionnaire (MPQ) EXCEPT that

    (A) it uses words to describe the sensory qualities of the pain experience
    (B) it uses words to describe the affective qualities of the pain experience
    (C) it describes subjective overall intensity of the total pain experience
    (D) it may be useful in identifying patients with suicidal ideation
    (E) it may be useful in discriminating between patients with functional versus organic causes of pain

274. True statements about the Minnesota Multiphasic Personality Inventory (MMPI) include which of the following?

    (A) It reliably discriminates between organic and psychogenic pain
    (B) It can predict the outcome in multimodal pain management programs
    (C) It can be used as the sole psychological test to measure coping strategies in patients with chronic pain
    (D) It may reveal a "conversion V" pattern in patients with chronic pain

PAIN MANAGEMENT

DIRECTIONS: Each question below contains four suggested responses of which **one or more** is correct. Select

A	if	**1, 2, and 3**	are correct
B	if	**1 and 3**	are correct
C	if	**2 and 4**	are correct
D	if	**4**	is correct
E	if	**1, 2, 3, and 4**	are correct

275. True statements regarding the Visual Analogue Scale (VAS) include which of the following?

    (1) A new VAS should be used at each evaluation
    (2) It is sensitive to pharmacologic procedures that alter experience of pain
    (3) It correlates highly with pain measured in verbal and numerical rating scales
    (4) It can be reliably administered by asking the patient to rate the amount or percentage of pain relief they have obtained from a therapeutic intervention

276. The Illness Behavior Assessment Schedule is

    (1) a test taken by patients with chronic pain to determine which treatments will benefit them
    (2) an assessment tool that can help to determine the extent to which somatic illness is being used defensively
    (3) an assessment tool that has shown that chronic abnormal illness behavior should be regarded as a form of depressive illness
    (4) a structured interview that allows the clinician to evaluate various components of illness behavior

277. The Illness Behavior Questionnaire is correctly characterized by which of the following statements?

    (1) It identifies organic causes of pain
    (2) It requires comments or essays to be written in response to questions
    (3) It takes approximately 1 to 2 h to complete
    (4) It provides scores on seven scales that assess the patient's attitudes and feelings about illness

278. Which of the following are considered positive outcomes of treatment in multidisciplinary pain management centers?

    (1) Diminished dependence on the health care system
    (2) Decreased consumption of medication
    (3) Increased gainful activities of daily living
    (4) Decreased pain scores on numeric rating scales

Pain Assessment

Answers

271. **The answer is C.** (*Bonica, pp 582–584.*) The McGill Pain Questionnaire (MPQ) is a widely used tool in the evaluation of pain. It has four main sections. The first section asks, "Where is your pain?" The patient is asked to mark an anatomic diagram and to also note whether the pain is experienced as internal, external, or both. The second section asks, "What does your pain feel like?" There are 20 categories of descriptors. The patient is asked to select the description from each category that best categorizes the pain. Categories 1 through 8 are sensory; 9 through 15 are affective; 16 is evaluative; and 17 through 20 are miscellaneous. The third section asks, "How does your pain change with time?" The fourth section asks, "How strong is your pain?" Analysis of the MPQ reveals that the total score is valid as a general measure of pain severity. Individual scale scores are not consistently valid. It does provide information about the sensory and affective components of the pain, making it a multidimensional tool that enriches understanding of pain as it impacts upon the individual patient.

272. **The answer is E.** (*Bonica, pp 581–582.*) The VAS is used to measure pain intensity at the time the scale is being marked. The distance in centimeters from the left to the patient's mark is the numerical index of the intensity of the patient's pain. Comparison with prior VASs of the patient provides a reliable and valid measure of the pain's intensity and its change over time.

273. **The answer is D.** (*Wall, pp 339–347.*) The MPQ is a reliable and reproducible test that can provide the pain-control practitioner with important information as to the physical and emotional experience of the patient. It has also been shown that each type of pain is characterized by a specific subset of descriptors on the MPQ. This may be helpful in differential diagnosis. In addition, patients with physical (organic) causes of pain select distinctly different words than those suffering from pain with no identifiable physical cause (functional). There is no particular descriptive pattern that identifies the suicidal patient.

274. **The answer is D.** (*Raj, pp 122–125. Tollison, pp 572–577. Wall, p 905.*) The MMPI (635 questions) does not reliably distinguish between psychogenic and physical (organic) pain, nor can it consistently predict the outcome of multimodal pain therapy. The conversion V is often present in patients with chronic pain:

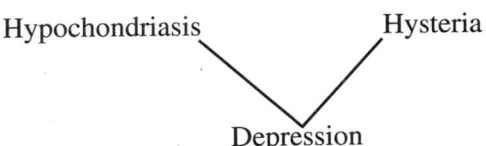

The conversion V has been shown to improve with treatment. Supplemental tests, such as the coping strategies questionnaire, should be used in conjunction with the MMPI. Other psychometric tests include the Symptoms-Checklist 90 in which the patient rates physical and emotional distress on a 5-point scale.

275. The answer is A (1,2,3). (*Wall, pp 338–339.*) The VAS provides a simple measurement of pain intensity. It does not characterize the complex pain experience. A new VAS should be used at each evaluation (so no bias can be introduced by what was marked before). The VAS is quite sensitive and reproducible. It correlates highly with verbal and numerical scales and is very sensitive to both pharmacologic and nonpharmacologic interventions that alter pain intensity. One should avoid asking for a "percentage of improvement" because this decreases the objective validity of the VAS.

276. The answer is C (2,4). (*Bonica, pp 304–305.*) Patients with chronic pain should undergo a comprehensive history and psychosocial evaluation as part of the initial admission for treatment in comprehensive programs of pain treatment. Various assessment tools may be helpful in providing insight into the patient's response to pain and coping mechanisms available to the patient. The Illness Behavior Assessment Schedule is a structured interview between the clinician and patient that allows the clinician to assess many psychosocial factors that contribute to abnormal illness behavior. It has been shown to be valid and reliable. The assessment tool is used to determine the patient's extent of understanding of the somatic illness as a cause of pain, disease conviction, symptom awareness, disease phobia, preoccupation with disease, illness-cause beliefs, communication of feelings, anxiety, depression, affective disturbance or denial of life's problems, and irritability. The assessment will help provide insight into the treatment approaches that may benefit the patient but does not definitively identify the best treatment plan by itself. In addition, studies indicate that chronic pain behavior should not be considered as a form of depressive illness, but that reactive depression may be a consequence of chronic pain and become a component of abnormal illness behavior.

277. The answer is D (4). (*Bonica, pp 304–307.*) The Illness Behavior Questionnaire (IBQ) consists of 62 questions to be answered "yes" or "no." It is not the same as the Illness Behavior Assessment Schedule, which is completed by the clinician after an extensive interview with the patient. The IBQ can be completed by most people in less than 30 min. It is used as a screening instrument that provides scores on seven scales that assess the patient's feelings about illness, affect, and attribution style. The scales are general hypochondriasis, disease conviction, psychological versus somatic perception of illness, affective inhibition, affective disturbance, denial, and irritability. The results are fairly reliable and valid and can be used to further explore other psychological issues during treatment.

278. The answer is E (all). (*Tollison, pp 656–663.*) Any comprehensive program of pain treatment should have a way of measuring effectiveness of therapy and assessing outcomes. Many different approaches have been recommended. Whichever method is chosen, it should include assessment of increases in gainful activities of daily living. Other positive outcomes include decreased consumption of medication, lower pain level as documented by numeric rating scales or other reliable assessment tools, changes in disability status, decreased use of the health care system, increased independence, and return to employment.

Pharmacology

DIRECTIONS: Each question below contains suggested responses. Select the **one best** response.

279. All the following are true statements regarding acetaminophen EXCEPT

    (A) it has analgesic properties similar to those of aspirin
    (B) it does not interfere with platelet function
    (C) it does not produce gastric irritation
    (D) its antipyretic effect is due to peripheral vasodilation
    (E) it is a paraaminophenol derivative

280. The mechanism of action through which methocarbamol produces muscle relaxation involves

    (A) receptor binding at the motor end plate
    (B) inhibition of nerve fiber conduction
    (C) depression of the central nervous system
    (D) blocking reuptake of acetylcholine
    (E) direct action on skeletal muscle

281. A 75-year-old dialysis patient underwent exploratory laparoscopy and lysis of adhesions. You are asked to recommend an appropriate postoperative analgesic regimen. Of the following, which is the best treatment option?

    (A) PCA morphine
    (B) PCA meperidine
    (C) IM ketorolac
    (D) Transdermal fentanyl
    (E) PCA hydromorphone

282. All the following are possible side effects of carbamazepine EXCEPT

    (A) vertigo
    (B) thrombocytopenia
    (C) hypertension
    (D) diplopia
    (E) gingival hyperplasia

283. After a single application of a Duragesic (transdermal fentanyl system) patch, peak serum concentrations will occur at

    (A) 4 to 8 h
    (B) 8 to 12 h
    (C) 12 to 18 h
    (D) 18 to 24 h
    (E) 24 to 72 h

284. The major obstacle to diffusion of fentanyl in the Duragesic patch is the

    (A) stratum corneum
    (B) dermis
    (C) hairy skin
    (D) subcutaneous fat
    (E) body temperature

285. The most appropriate nonsteroidal anti-inflammatory drug (NSAID) to use in a lactating female is

(A) piroxicam
(B) diflunisal
(C) ketorolac
(D) naproxen
(E) ibuprofen

286. The following statements regarding drug interactions with NSAIDs are true EXCEPT that

(A) NSAIDs prolong the prothrombin time (PT) in patients on warfarin
(B) the combination of diflunisal and indomethacin has resulted in fatal gastric hemorrhage
(C) inhibition of platelet aggregation by NSAIDs makes the patient more susceptible to bleeding
(D) There is less risk of gastrointestinal (GI) adverse effects in patients taking steroids
(E) misoprostol has been shown to prevent NSAID-induced gastropathy

287. Select the statement that best describes the action of NSAIDs.

(A) NSAIDs have their main activity in the CNS
(B) Tolerance may occur with long-term use
(C) NSAIDs are potent cyclooxygenase inhibitors
(D) NSAIDs facilitate neutrophil migration and lymphocyte responsiveness

288. Which of the following statements is true of acetaminophen?

(A) It is less potent than aspirin as an analgesic
(B) It is more potent than aspirin as an antipyretic
(C) It is a weak anti-inflammatory
(D) A dose of 1500 mg will provide significantly greater analgesia than 1000 mg
(E) It is well tolerated by patients with alcoholic liver damage

289. Which of the following is implicated in the production of morphine-induced pain?

(A) Morphine-6-glucuronide
(B) Morphine hydrochloride
(C) Diacetylmorphine
(D) Morphine-3-glucuronide
(E) 6-Monoacetylmorphine

290. A 27-year-old man who had been taking two Percocet tablets (oxycodone and acetaminophen) every 4 h for the last 2 months came in to the ER complaining of abdominal cramps, nausea, and vomiting. Upon further questioning, he states that the Percocet tablets were making him nauseated and therefore he recently changed to extra-strength Tylenol (acetaminophen). The nausea initially improved, but then increased significantly over the last 24 to 48 h. No one else in his family is ill. His evaluation in the ER revealed no other abnormalities except for a heart rate of 105 beats per minute. What is the most likely cause of this patient's GI distress?

(A) Addiction to Percocet
(B) Tolerance to Percocet
(C) Side effects of Percocet
(D) Physical dependence on Percocet
(E) Viral influenza

291. Which of the following drugs is most preferred for treatment of cancer pain?

(A) Buprenorphine
(B) Cannabinoids
(C) Meperidine
(D) Levorphanol
(E) Butorphanol

292. Which of the following statements best describes the action of a specific drug at opioid receptor sites?

(A) Naltrexone acts as an antagonist at mu but not kappa receptor sites
(B) Butorphanol has no action at the sigma receptor site
(C) Pentazocine is a partial agonist at the kappa receptor site and an antagonist at the mu receptor
(D) Morphine does not act at the kappa receptor
(E) Buprenorphine is a sigma receptor antagonist

293. Early signs of local anesthetic toxicity after intravenous administration include all the following EXCEPT

(A) tinnitus
(B) hypotension
(C) agitation
(D) metallic taste
(E) light-headedness

294. Which of the following factors has a significant effect on the distribution of local anesthetic in CSF?

(A) Composition of CSF
(B) Concentration of injected local anesthetic
(C) Addition of vasoconstrictors to the local anesthetic
(D) Site of injection
(E) Patient weight

295. A hyperbaric local anesthetic solution would have a specific gravity of

(A) 1.0010
(B) 1.0008
(C) 1.0003
(D) 0.9990
(E) 0.9950

296. Which of the following antidepressants has the LEAST anticholingeric and sedating effects?

(A) Amitriptyline (Elavil)
(B) Imipramine (Tofranil)
(C) Desipramine (Norpramin)
(D) Doxepin (Sinequan)

297. A 50-year-old man with chronic low back pain and a history of heart block was started on a tricyclic antidepressant (TCA). Which drug would be the most appropriate choice?

(A) Trazodone (Desyrel)
(B) Desipramine (Norpramin)
(C) Amitriptyline (Elavil)
(D) Nortriptyline (Pamelor)

298. Which of the following antidepressant medications is considered the LEAST cardiotoxic?

(A) Doxepin (Sinequan)
(B) Trazodone (Desyrel)
(C) Nortriptyline (Pamelor)
(D) Desipramine (Norpramin)

299. All the following statements about aspirin hypersensitivity are true EXCEPT that

(A) it occurs most commonly in middle-aged adults
(B) it is more common in females
(C) it has no cross-sensitivity to other NSAIDs
(D) it is not classified as a true allergic reaction
(E) it usually occurs within minutes of taking aspirin

300. Symptoms associated with the administration of interferon include all the following EXCEPT

(A) fever and chills
(B) tenesmus and diarrhea
(C) myalgias and arthralgias
(D) headache

301. A cancer patient undergoing a rapid infusion of 100 mg of dexamethasone complains of an intense burning sensation in the perineum after the injection. The most likely cause of this symptom is

(A) anxiety reaction
(B) tumor metastasis
(C) steroid psychosis
(D) drug-related side effect

302. Which of the following antidepressants is the LEAST sedating?

(A) Amitriptyline (Elavil)
(B) Doxepin (Sinequan)
(C) Trazodone (Desyrel)
(D) Desipramine (Norpramin)

303. In general, all antidepressants

(A) are hydrophilic
(B) are poorly absorbed in the GI tract
(C) have extensive first-pass hepatic metabolism
(D) are poorly bound to alpha-1 acid glycoprotein

304. All the following medications have been associated with muscle cramps EXCEPT

(A) phenothiazines
(B) lithium
(C) cimetidine
(D) diazepam

305. The addition of epinephrine to lidocaine

    (A) speeds absorption and increases peak blood levels
    (B) prolongs the action of lidocaine
    (C) has no effect on systemic toxicity
    (D) causes local vasodilation

306. Which of the following statements is true regarding opioid-induced constipation?

    (A) Itching and nausea are much more common side effects than constipation
    (B) Tolerance develops to the constipating effects of opioids
    (C) Bowel obstruction has not occurred with the use of high-dose opioids
    (D) The patient should be placed on a regular regimen of laxatives and stool softeners from the start of opioid therapy

307. Morphine 10 mg intramuscularly (IM) has roughly the same analgesic potency as

    (A) 200 mg codeine IM
    (B) 2 mg levorphanol (Levo-Dromoran) IM
    (C) 200 mg meperidine (Demerol) IM
    (D) 5 mg methadone IM

308. Which of the following statements is true regarding the use of antidepressants as analgesics?

    (A) The analgesic effect is primarily due to the relief of depression
    (B) The antidepressants have no analgesic effect in patients who do not have depression
    (C) To obtain analgesia, a trial of at least 6 months is needed
    (D) Analgesic response usually occurs at a lower dose than that required for treatment of clinical depression

309. Which of the following local anesthetics is NOT recommended for use in tissue infiltration?

    (A) Procaine
    (B) Tetracaine
    (C) Lidocaine
    (D) Bupivacaine

310. Which of the following drugs is an amino ester local anesthetic?

    (A) Etidocaine
    (B) Ropivacaine
    (C) Mepivacaine
    (D) Tetracaine

311. Which of the following drugs, if given within 10 h of an overdose of acetaminophen, may protect the liver from lethal injury?

    (A) Sodium acetylcysteine
    (B) Amiodarone
    (C) Sodium valproate
    (D) Prednisone

312. A 50-year-old man has been taking 6 to 10 acetaminophen tablets supplemented by 4 to 6 aspirin tablets daily for over 3 years as treatment for his chronic low back pain. On routine physical examination and testing he was found to have a serum creatinine of 3.2, a hematocrit of 27, blood pressure of 160/100, and heart rate of 80 beats per minute. What is the most appropriate treatment for this patient?

    (A) Immediate hemodialysis
    (B) Blood transfusion
    (C) Stopping acetaminophen and aspirin
    (D) Administration of acetylcysteine

313. Which of the following is true regarding placebo analgesia?

    (A) Placebo analgesics are drugs that were originally used to treat another disease process and were coincidentally found to have analgesic properties
    (B) Patients receiving placebos do not report the side effects often associated with non-placebo drugs
    (C) The expected response rate to placebo analgesia in any large study would be 10 percent
    (D) The personality of the patient and cultural attitudes about pain play a part in the placebo response
    (E) Tolerance and the occurrence of abstinence syndrome have not been documented to occur in patients receiving placebo analgesia

PHARMACOLOGY

314. All the following are analgesic adjuvants EXCEPT

    (A) caffeine
    (B) dextroamphetamine
    (C) tricyclic antidepressants
    (D) hydroxyzine
    (E) metoclopramide

315. Preventive treatment of cluster headaches includes

    (A) daytime napping
    (B) small amounts of alcohol for relaxation
    (C) low-dose narcotic analgesics
    (D) prednisone
    (E) sumatriptan

316. Which of the following is true regarding absorption rate of local anesthetic after nerve block?

    (A) Caudal block is greater than epidural block
    (B) Femoral nerve block is greater than brachial plexus block
    (C) Caudal block is greater than intercostal block
    (D) Epidural block is greater than intercostal block
    (E) Brachial plexus block is greater than caudal block

317. Which of the following is a pharmacodynamic activity of a drug?

    (A) Absorption
    (B) Receptor binding
    (C) Metabolism
    (D) Distribution

318. Which of the following general statements is true regarding the protein binding of drugs?

    (A) The protein-bound drug is the active drug
    (B) Albumin is the least important protein-binding site
    (C) Alpha-1 acid glycoprotein binds primarily acidic drugs
    (D) The volume of distribution is inversely related to protein binding

319. All the following medications may cause drug-induced depression EXCEPT

    (A) oral contraceptives
    (B) propranolol
    (C) high-dose steroids
    (D) opioids

320. Which antidepressant has the highest risk of inducing seizures?

    (A) Doxepine (Sinequan)
    (B) Trazodone (Desyrel)
    (C) Amitriptyline (Elavil)
    (D) Maprotiline (Ludiomil)

321. Which antidepressant has the greatest risk of causing significant extrapyramidal symptoms?

    (A) Desipramine (Norpramin)
    (B) Amoxapine (Asendin)
    (C) Imipramine (Tofranil)
    (D) Fluoxetine (Prozac)

322. With the use of this specific drug, hypotension is common, especially in patients whose blood pressure is already low. Priapism occurs in approximately 1 out of 1000 males. There may be an increased incidence of ventricular arrhythmias in patients with preexisting cardiac disease.
    The above constellation of side effects best describes which of the following drugs?

    (A) Amitriptyline (Elavil)
    (B) Doxepin (Sinequan)
    (C) Trazodone (Desyrel)
    (D) Venlafaxine (Effexor)

323. A 40-year-old patient with chronic low back pain was taking 125 mg doxepin (Sinequan) PO every night for 4 weeks. He did not note any benefit from the medication and decided to stop taking it. The evening after discontinuing the doxepin, the patient had vivid dreams and awoke in the morning with a headache. He also had diarrhea. What is the most likely etiology of his new complaints?

    (A) He ate something that did not agree with him for dinner the night before
    (B) He is developing early signs of viral influenza
    (C) He is going through mild withdrawal reactions
    (D) He is having an anxiety reaction

324. In open label studies of the treatment of central poststroke pain, which of the following drugs was found to enhance the effectiveness of doxepin?

    (A) Venlafaxine (Effexor)
    (B) Terbutaline (Bricanyl)
    (C) Propranolol (Inderal)
    (D) Acetaminophen (Tylenol)

325. Which of the following accurately describes strontium-89?

    (A) It is useful for treatment of painful bony metastases in patients with prostatic or breast cancer
    (B) It must be injected intraarterially to be effective
    (C) It does not suppress the bone marrow
    (D) It emits both beta and gamma radiation

326. A relative contraindication to the use of botulinum A toxin is

    (A) strabismus
    (B) myofascial pain for greater than 6 months
    (C) spasticity after spinal cord injury
    (D) myasthenia gravis
    (E) use of tricylcic antidepressants

327. All the following statements regarding botulinum A toxin are true EXCEPT

    (A) it inhibits the release of acetylcholine
    (B) it must enter the nerve endings to exert its effect
    (C) it is produced by *Clostridium botulinum*
    (D) its effect on the neuromuscular junction is not permanent
    (E) its clinical effect can be seen within 1 h after injection

328. Which of the following statements is true regarding the use of lithium in a hyponatremic patient?

    (A) More lithium is required to achieve a therapeutic effect
    (B) Sodium balance has no effect on lithium clearance
    (C) Metabolism of lithium is increased
    (D) Renal lithium excretion is reduced

329. All the following medications have been used for successful treatment of the symptoms of erythromelalgia EXCEPT

    (A) acetylsalicylic acid (aspirin)
    (B) phenoxybenzamine (Dibenzyline)
    (C) methysergide (Sansert)
    (D) diphenylhydantoin (Dilantin)

330. Which of the following may decrease the efficacy of intravenous regional blockade with guanethidine?

    (A) Cimetidine
    (B) Amitriptyline
    (C) Steroids
    (D) Tobacco

331. Which local anesthetic can cause methemoglobinemia?

    (A) Bupivacaine
    (B) Lidocaine
    (C) Prilocaine
    (D) Tetracaine

332. Which of the following statements is true regarding addictive behavior in the chronic pain population?

    (A) Drug addiction is more common in chronic pain patients than in general society
    (B) The prevalence of drug abuse, dependence, or addiction is less than 20 percent in the chronic pain population
    (C) Because of the high incidence of addiction, opioid use is contraindicated in chronic pain patients
    (D) Alcohol abuse is more common in chronic pain patients than in general society

333. Lithium for pain control is contraindicated in patients with all the following medical conditions EXCEPT

    (A) myasthenia gravis
    (B) renal tubular disease
    (C) cardiac conduction defects
    (D) depression

334. What is the shortest-acting opioid?

    (A) Butorphanol
    (B) Meperidine
    (C) Morphine
    (D) MS-Contin

335. Which of the following is true regarding corticosteroids?

    (A) They have potent analgesic properties
    (B) They help to prevent destruction of joints
    (C) Methylprednisolone is a long-acting corticosteroid
    (D) They are potent anti-inflammatory agents

336. The approximate dose equivalents to 10 mg of morphine are

    (A) 100 mg meperidine, 25 μg fentanyl, 500 μg alfentanil, 5 mg methadone
    (B) 100 mg meperidine, 100 μg fentanyl, 500 μg alfentanil, 10 mg methadone
    (C) 50 mg meperidine, 50 μg fentanyl, 500 μg alfentanil, 5 mg methadone
    (D) 50 mg meperidine, 100 μg fentanyl, 250 μg alfentanil, 10 mg methadone

337. What is the most appropriate medication for the treatment of benzodiazepine withdrawal?

    (A) Morphine
    (B) Clonidine
    (C) Tricyclic antidepressants
    (D) Phenobarbital
    (E) Diazepam

338. Which of the following is true regarding withdrawal from short-acting opioids?

    (A) Seizures may occur
    (B) Withdrawal is often life-threatening
    (C) Withdrawal symptoms peak at 48 to 72 h
    (D) Untreated withdrawal resolves in 3 to 5 days
    (E) Sedation and hypersomnia occur at the peak of withdrawal

339. Which local anesthetic is most likely to be associated with an allergic reaction?

    (A) Mepivacaine
    (B) Bupivacaine
    (C) Lidocaine
    (D) Tetracaine
    (E) Ropivacaine

340. All the following are true statements about intravenous phentolamine EXCEPT

    (A) phentolamine is a short-acting, competitive, alpha-adrenergic antagonist
    (B) intravenous phentolamine has been used as a test to diagnose reflex sympathetic dystrophy
    (C) intravenous phentolamine is equally effective in relieving stimulus-independent and stimulus-evoked pain
    (D) there should be a marked increase in skin temperature of the painful extremity in the intravenous phentolamine test as there is with lumbar sympathetic block
    (E) the pain-reducing effect of intravenous phentolamine is peripheral, not central

PAIN MANAGEMENT

DIRECTIONS: Each question below contains four suggested responses of which **one or more** is correct. Select

A	if	**1, 2, and 3**	are correct
B	if	**1 and 3**	are correct
C	if	**2 and 4**	are correct
D	if	**4**	is correct
E	if	**1, 2, 3, and 4**	are correct

341. Nonacetylated salicylates include
    (1) salsalate
    (2) diflunisal
    (3) choline magnesium trisalicylate
    (4) sulindac

342. True statements regarding tolerance include that it
    (1) is characteristic of opioids as a class
    (2) cannot occur without physical dependence
    (3) is defined as requiring more drug to produce the same effect
    (4) is synonymous with addiction

343. Opioid antagonists include
    (1) naltrexone
    (2) cholecystokinin
    (3) naloxone
    (4) dezocine

344. Clinical properties of opioid agonist-antagonists and partial agonists include
    (1) lower potency than pure agonists
    (2) lower addiction potential than morphine
    (3) ceiling effect for both respiratory depression and analgesia
    (4) dysphoric reactions

345. Opioids that cause histamine release include
    (1) meperidine
    (2) sufentanil
    (3) codeine
    (4) fentanyl

346. Symptomatic treatment of cluster headaches includes
    (1) cyproheptadine
    (2) ergotamine
    (3) Bellergal (combination of phenobarbital, ergotamine, and levorotatory alkaloids of belladonna)
    (4) oxygen

347. Statements that correctly characterize clonidine include that
    (1) it inhibits nociceptive neurons in the dorsal horn
    (2) it is an alpha$_1$ agonist
    (3) it produces analgesia when applied to the spinal cord in animals
    (4) it does not produce analgesia when applied to the spinal cord in humans

348. Tachyphylaxis with a local anesthetic is
    (1) more likely to occur when a drug is administered by intermittent boluses than when given continuously
    (2) associated with a shorter duration of action and fading anesthetic potency
    (3) less likely with the addition of acidic antioxidants to the solution
    (4) defined as a drug's declining effectiveness when given repeatedly

349. Which of the following can cause severe drug-induced myalgia?
    (1) Trazodone
    (2) Amphetamines
    (3) Acetaminophen
    (4) Alcohol

350. Compared with morphine, buprenorphine
    (1) is more potent
    (2) is more lipid-soluble
    (3) has a greater affinity for opioid receptors
    (4) is less protein-bound

PHARMACOLOGY

351. A 35-year-old woman with breast cancer and metastatic lesions to ribs and lumbar spine presents to the ER with slowly increasing, severe pain. Over the last 2 months, she has been taking controlled-release morphine sulfate (MS-Contin) 90 mg bid and ibuprofen 600 mg qid. After extensive evaluation revealed no new metastases or CNS pathology, which oral medications below would be appropriate to add to her current regimen?

    (1) Increased MS-Contin
    (2) Amitriptyline 25 mg qhs
    (3) Increased ibuprofen to 800 mg qid
    (4) Pentazocine for breakthrough pain

352. True statements regarding naproxen include that

    (1) peak plasma concentrations occur within 2 h after an oral dose
    (2) it is an acetic acid derivative
    (3) it is extensively bound to plasma proteins
    (4) it has an elimination half-life of 4 to 6 h

353. True statements regarding epidural opioids include that

    (1) they bind to epidural fat
    (2) they enter the systemic circulation by way of the epidural venous system
    (3) they reach the dorsal horn by way of the posterior radicular arteries
    (4) they enter the cerebrospinal fluid (CSF) through the dura by diffusing across arachnoid granulations

354. Fentanyl-induced pruritus has been treated by

    (1) butorphanol
    (2) buprenorphine
    (3) nalbuphine
    (4) levorphanol

355. In comparison to alcohol, phenol

    (1) produces a less profound block
    (2) deteriorates in storage after 1 month
    (3) produces a block of shorter duration
    (4) is hypobaric

356. Complications resulting from bolus injections of local anesthetic into the internal carotid artery include

    (1) aphasia
    (2) convulsions
    (3) hemiparesis
    (4) total blindness

357. Intravascular injection of 10% phenol can cause

    (1) flushing
    (2) a pleasurable sensation
    (3) severe tinnitus
    (4) thrombosis

358. The most important factors in determining the spread of spinal anesthetic solutions include

    (1) volume of anesthetic injected
    (2) baricity of the anesthetic solution
    (3) position of the patient
    (4) addition of vasoconstrictors to the solution

359. True statements regarding methylparaben include that

    (1) it is an antimicrobial agent added to some local anesthetic solutions
    (2) it is typically used as a 10% solution
    (3) it may be responsible for allergic reactions attributed to local anesthetics
    (4) it is most effective against gram-negative organisms

360. Headache may occur after the administration of which of the following antineoplastic agents?

    (1) Intrathecal methotrexate
    (2) L-Asparaginase
    (3) Transretinoic acid
    (4) 5-Fluorouracil

361. There is an increased risk of anticholinergic delirium when amitriptyline is used in conjunction with which of the following medications?

    (1) Phenothiazines
    (2) Atropine
    (3) Diphenhydramine
    (4) Meperidine

SUMMARY OF DIRECTIONS				
A	B	C	D	E
1,2,3 only	1,3 only	2,4 only	4 only	All are correct

362. Selective serotonin reuptake inhibitors (SSRIs) include

    (1) fluoxetine (Prozac)
    (2) maprotiline (Ludiomil)
    (3) sertraline (Zoloft)
    (4) venlafaxine (Effexor)

363. Chemotherapeutic agents known to cause mental status changes include which of the following drugs?

    (1) Methotrexate
    (2) Vincristine
    (3) Bleomycin
    (4) 5-Fluorouracil

364. A 40-year-old woman had been taking 50 mg of baclofen (Lioresal) each day for the last 6 months for the treatment of spasticity associated with multiple sclerosis. She then developed viral gastroenteritis, which prevented her from taking baclofen for over 24 h. The patient should be observed for which of the following symptoms after this abrupt withdrawal of baclofen?

    (1) Coma
    (2) Hallucinations
    (3) Stroke
    (4) Seizures

365. The placebo effect is correctly characterized by which of the following?

    (1) It occurs when an intervention that is not expected to have an effect produces one
    (2) It occurs in over 30 percent of the population in the case of analgesia
    (3) It mandates a double-blind crossover study design
    (4) It can be measured using sophisticated psychological testing

366. True statements about the "nocebo" effect include

    (1) effects are commonly the same as expected from the active agent
    (2) it implies the presence of psychogenic pain
    (3) it occurs when ineffective interventions produce adverse effects
    (4) the McGill Pain Questionnaire is used to predict its occurrence

367. Factors that predispose to the development of late-onset respiratory depression following administration of spinal opioids include

    (1) large doses of opioids
    (2) thoracic epidural opioids
    (3) opioid-naive patients
    (4) use of lipid-soluble opioids

368. Physiologic properties of the body affecting the volume of distribution of a drug include

    (1) local pH
    (2) tissue composition
    (3) membrane permeability
    (4) blood flow

369. Drugs used to prevent migraine include

    (1) beta blockers
    (2) methysergide
    (3) cyproheptadine
    (4) lithium

370. Medications used in the symptomatic treatment of migraine include

    (1) ergotamine tartrate
    (2) isometheptene mucate
    (3) meclofenamate sodium
    (4) sumatriptan

371. Physiochemical properties of a drug that influence its volume of distribution include

    (1) molecular weight
    (2) lipid solubility
    (3) degree of ionization
    (4) polarity

PHARMACOLOGY

372. Allergic reactions to local anesthetics
    (1) are less common with the addition of methylparaben
    (2) are frequently misdiagnosed as systemic toxic reactions
    (3) occur more commonly with the amino-amide agents
    (4) may involve para-aminobenzoic acid

373. The development of tachyphylaxis
    (1) is affected by the concentration of local anesthetic used
    (2) occurs with continuous infusion as well as intermittent boluses of local anesthetic
    (3) has been well documented to occur with both lidocaine and bupivacaine
    (4) occurs more often in patients receiving combined local anesthetic and opioid mixtures epidurally

374. Phenol in glycerin, a commonly used subarachnoid neurolytic agent,
    (1) is less painful on injection compared with alcohol
    (2) is hyperbaric compared with the CSF
    (3) causes nonselective destruction of nervous tissue
    (4) produces neurolysis by causing protein degeneration

375. True statements regarding the injection of glycerol include
    (1) it is injected into the trigeminal ganglion for treatment of trigeminal neuralgia
    (2) topical application is more damaging than intraneural injection
    (3) wallerian degeneration occurs
    (4) regeneration begins within 1 month of injection

376. Calcitonin has been used as an effective analgesic in which of the following conditions?
    (1) Phantom limb pain
    (2) Paget's disease
    (3) Bony metastases
    (4) Osteoarthritis

377. Botulinum A toxin is an effective treatment in which of the following conditions?
    (1) Strabismus
    (2) Myofascial pain
    (3) Blepharospasm
    (4) Torticollis

378. Agents that may be beneficial to AIDS patients with painful sensory neuropathy include
    (1) tricyclic antidepressants
    (2) carbamazepine
    (3) topical capsaicin
    (4) opioid analgesics

379. Psychological dependence (addiction) is characterized by
    (1) craving for drug effects other than pain relief
    (2) persistent efforts to obtain sufficient narcotic to control pain
    (3) tendency to relapse after withdrawal
    (4) withdrawal symptoms when the drug is withheld

380. Which of the following may increase the clearance of other drugs?
    (1) Smoking
    (2) Phenytoin
    (3) Barbiturates
    (4) Cimetidine

381. Risks associated with chronic use of corticosteroids include
    (1) osteoporosis
    (2) avascular necrosis of bone
    (3) hypertension
    (4) cataract formation

382. Which of the following medications can be used as treatment for opioid withdrawal?
    (1) Clonidine
    (2) Diphenylhydantoin
    (3) Buprenorphine
    (4) Phenobarbital

PAIN MANAGEMENT

SUMMARY OF DIRECTIONS				
A	B	C	D	E
1,2,3 only	1,3 only	2,4 only	4 only	All are correct

383. Appropriate medications for management of the symptoms of alcohol withdrawal include

    (1) lorazepam
    (2) buprenorphine
    (3) diazepam
    (4) clonidine

384. How does alkalinization of urine affect the elimination of tricyclic antidepressants?

    (1) Metabolism is increased
    (2) Excretion rate is decreased
    (3) Clearance rate is not affected
    (4) Reabsorption is increased

Pharmacology

Answers

279. The answer is D. (*Raj, p 610.*) Acetaminophen is a paraaminophenol derivative with analgesic and antipyretic properties similar to those of aspirin. The antipyretic effect appears to result from a direct action on the hypothalamic heat-regulating center. However, the peripheral prostaglandin synthetase inhibition noted with aspirin is not found with acetaminophen. Acetaminophen neither interferes with platelet function nor causes gastric irritation.

280. The answer is C. (*Physicians' Desk Reference [PDR], 1995, pp 2014–2015.*) Methocarbamol is a skeletal muscle relaxant that is indicated for the relief of discomfort associated with acute, painful musculoskeletal conditions. The mechanism of action is thought to be depression of the central nervous system. Methocarbamol does not have any direct action on the contractile mechanism of striated muscle, the motor end plate, or the nerve fiber.

281. The answer is E. (*Ferrante, pp 138–139, 172–173, 176–181. Raj, pp 623, 626, 627.*) There are multiple medical problems associated with renal failure. Meperidine undergoes transformation to normeperidine, which has a long half-life and may accumulate, especially in patients with renal failure. Normeperidine has been associated with CNS irritability syndrome (myoclonus and seizures may occur). Morphine has an active metabolite, morphine 6-glucuronide. Elimination of this metabolite is impaired in patients with renal dysfunction, and accumulation of morphine 6-glucuronide can cause increased sedation. Fentanyl has no active metabolites. There is no prolongation in the elimination rate in patients with renal dysfunction. PCA fentanyl would be useful in patients with renal failure. However, in patch-form, the fentanyl concentration increases over 12 to 18 h until a steady state is reached. Once the patch is removed, the concentration will slowly decrease, with a half-life of 15 to 21 h. Therefore, the dosage is difficult to titrate to maximally treat acute pain. Ketorolac has not been shown to have direct nephrotoxic effects. However, all NSAIDs inhibit prostaglandins, which in turn can decrease renal blood flow. In addition, IM injection is painful and there may be an increased risk of IM bleeding in uremic patients. Ketorolac has recently been approved for intravenous administration. Hydromorphone has no active metabolites, making it a useful drug for patients with renal failure.

282. The answer is E. (*Stoelting, pp 501–503.*) Nausea, vomiting, sedation, vertigo, diplopia, and ataxia are the most common side effects of carbamazepine therapy. Other potentially life-threatening side effects include aplastic anemia, thrombocytopenia, hepatocellular and cholestatic jaundice, oliguria, hypertension, and acute left ventricular failure. Gingival hyperplasia is a common side effect of chronic phenytoin therapy.

283. The answer is E. (*PDR, 1995, pp 1178–1181.*) Duragesic is a transdermal system providing continuous systemic delivery of fentanyl. The amount of fentanyl released from each system per hour is proportional to the surface area of the patch. Peak serum levels of fentanyl generally occur from 24 to 72 h after a single application of the patch.

284. **The answer is A.** (*Ferrante, p 181.*) The major obstacle to diffusion of fentanyl from a Duragesic patch is the stratum corneum. Diffusion occurs primarily via the intracellular lipid medium. The dermis acts as a reservoir that requires filling before sustained systemic absorption can occur. As the depot is established, absorption continues even when the patch is removed.

285. **The answer is E.** (*Wall, p 930.*) NSAIDs are generally not recommended for use in nursing mothers because of the possible adverse effects on the infant. If they are used in lactating females (e.g., for treatment of arthritis), the drug should be taken just before breast-feeding so that plasma levels are low. Drugs should be used that have short half-lives and whose metabolites are inert and rapidly metabolized. Two such NSAIDs that have been used successfully in lactating women are ibuprofen and flurbiprofen.

286. **The answer is D.** (*Wall, pp 926–927.*) NSAIDs prolong the PT in patients on warfarin by displacing it from protein-binding sites and thereby increasing the amount of free drug. Diflunisal and indomethacin decrease renal clearance, which significantly increases the levels of indomethacin. This has been associated with fatal gastric hemorrhage. Platelet aggregation is reversibly inhibited by most NSAIDs and will increase the risk of bleeding. After five half-lives, the drug will be almost completely eliminated, as will the antiplatelet effect. It is important to remember that platelets are irreversibly inhibited by aspirin. Its antiplatelet effect continues until the body has produced an adequate number of new platelets. Factors that increase the risk of adverse GI effects include age greater than 60 years, prior history of serious GI events, smoking, alcohol, concomitant use of anticoagulants or steroids, and high doses of NSAIDs. Misoprostol (Cytotec) is effective in preventing NSAID-induced gastropathy. H_2-receptor blockers have been effective in the presence of duodenal ulcers. NSAIDs taken with meals may have less GI effect. Antacids can decrease absorption of NSAIDs and decrease analgesic effectiveness.

287. **The answer is C.** (*Ferrante, p 134. Wall, p 923.*) NSAIDs have their main pharmacologic action in the periphery, though they have also been found to have some activity in the CNS. They do not bind to opioid receptor sites. Tolerance and physical dependence do not develop. There is a ceiling effect for analgesia (increasing the dose beyond a certain point does not increase analgesia). NSAIDs inhibit the enzyme cyclooxygenase (prostaglandin synthetase), which prevents arachidonic acid from being metabolized to the cyclic endoperoxides that produce thromboxane, prostaglandins, prostacyclin, and toxic oxygen radicals. NSAIDs also have nonprostaglandin-mediated effects such as inhibition of neutrophil migration and lymphocyte responsiveness.

288. **The answer is C.** (*Wall, pp 923–924.*) Acetaminophen is *equipotent* to aspirin as an analgesic and antipyretic but is a weak anti-inflammatory and has almost no antiplatelet effect. Its effects are thought to be through inhibition of brain prostaglandin synthetase. Patients with chronic alcoholism or liver damage may develop hepatotoxicity if they take acetaminophen, even at the prescribed doses. Acetaminophen overdose (25 g or more) can cause fatal hepatic necrosis. A ceiling effect for analgesia is reached at 1000 mg. The total daily dose should not exceed 4000 mg.

289. **The answer is D.** (*Wall, pp 952–953.*) When given at high doses, additional morphine may exacerbate rather than decrease pain. The mechanism by which this occurs is thought to be abnormal morphine metabolism. Morphine-6-glucuronide is more potent than morphine and may contribute to the analgesic effect of morphine. However, morphine-3-glucuronide antagonizes the effects of both morphine and morphine-6-glucuronide and may even be a direct, nonspecific cerebral stimulant. Seizures, myoclonus, and hyperalgesia have been documented to occur not only with high-dose morphine but also with fentanyl, hydromorphones, and other opioids.

290. **The answer is D.** (*Ferrante, p 165.*) This patient is suffering from abstinence syndrome (withdrawal) due to his physical dependence on Percocet. Symptoms of withdrawal include yawning, diaphoresis, lacrimation, coryza, tachycardia, abdominal cramps, nausea, and vomiting. Tolerance is the condition in which the continued use of opioids results in the requirement of increasing amounts of opioid to get the same analgesic

effect. All opioids eventually produce tolerance. There is incomplete cross-tolerance with other opioids. Tolerance can occur without physical dependence or addiction. Addiction is a psychological and sometimes physical state characterized by behaviors that include compulsion to take a particular drug in order to experience the psychic effects and sometimes to avoid the physical effects associated with abstinence.

291. The answer is D. (*Jacox, p 72.*) Butorphanol (a mixed agonist-antagonist) and buprenorphine (a partial agonist) have an analgesic ceiling and may precipitate withdrawal in patients on chronic opioid therapy. Cannabinoids have been used for analgesic and antiemetic effects. However, the side effects of dysphoria, drowsiness, hypotension and bradycardia are significant. Meperidine is a short-acting opioid agonist with potential for CNS toxicity such as tremor, confusion, and seizures, especially in patients with renal failure or with long-term use. Levorphanol is recommended by the AHCPR as one of the preferred opioids for treatment of cancer pain.

292. The answer is C. (*Ferrante, p 155.*) The following pharmacologic effects have been related to drug interactions at specific opioid receptors: mu—analgesia, respiratory depression, GI dysmotility, bradycardia; kappa—spinal analgesia, sedation; sigma—dysphoria. The table below shows the actions of particular drugs at receptor sites.

Drug	Receptor		
	Mu	Kappa	Sigma
Morphine	+	+	
Buprenorphine	±		
Dezocine	±		
Pentazocine	−	±	+
Nalbuphine	−	±	−
Butorphanol	−	±	+
Naloxone	−	−	−
Naltrexone	−	−	−

+ agonist; ± partial agonist; − antagonist

293. The answer is B. (*Cousins, p 922.*) Early signs and symptoms of local anesthetic toxicity include metallic taste, tinnitus, light-headedness, agitation, and drowsiness. Untoward effects of late CNS toxicity include hypotension or hypertension, bradycardia or tachycardia, seizures, and unconsciousness. Cardiac and respiratory failure, coma, and death may occur in the late stages of local anesthetic toxicity.

294. The answer is D. (*Cousins, p 224.*) When all the factors that affect distribution are kept constant, factors that have no demonstrable, significant effects on distribution of local anesthetic in CSF include patient weight, composition of CSF, CSF circulation, concentration of local anesthetic in the solution injected, diffusion of local anesthetics in CSF independent of the effects of baricity, addition of vasoconstrictor to the local anesthetic solution, and circulation of CSF. The site of injection, especially if at a level other than the L3–L4 interspace, is an important determinant of spread.

295. The answer is A. (*Cousins, pp 224-225.*) If the baricity of a solution is 1.0, it is by definition isobaric; if greater than 1.0, it is hyperbaric; and if less than 1.0, it is hypobaric. However, the density of normal CSF varies by 0.0003 (2 standard deviations) above and below the mean value of 1.0003. For spinal anesthetic solutions to be predictably hypobaric or hyperbaric in all patients requires that their baricities be, respectively, less than 0.9990 and greater than 1.0010.

296. The answer is C. (*Tollison, p 90.*) Anticholinergic, CNS, and cardiac side effects are more common with tertiary amines such as amitriptyline, imipramine, and doxepin, than with demethylated secondary amines (nortriptyline, desipramine). Desipramine is the least sedating and has the least anticholinergic effects of all the TCAs.

297. The answer is D. (*Tollison, p 90.*) Nortriptyline is less likely to depress AV conduction and less likely to produce orthostatic hypotension. It is the best choice for patients with bradyarrhythmias, heart block, or prolonged QT intervals. Doxepin (Sinequan) is also relatively noncardiotoxic. Imipramine (Tofranil) has been shown to suppress ventricular ectopy.

298. The answer is B. (*Wall, p 828.*) The second-generation antidepressants (e.g., trazodone) are considered less cardiotoxic than the tricyclic antidepressants (e.g., doxepin, nortriptyline, desipramine). Trazodone is very sedating. If given at bedtime, it can be used to facilitate sleep. It is also associated with a significant incidence of priapism and should be used cautiously in male patients.

299. The answer is C. (*Wall, p 925.*) Aspirin hypersensitivity usually occurs in middle-aged adults, more often in females. It is not classified as a true allergic reaction; the exact mechanism is unknown. There are two subgroups of aspirin-sensitive patients. In one subgroup, reaction is associated with rhinitis, asthma, or nasal polyps and is primarily respiratory. The other subtype develops wheals, angioneurotic edema, urticaria, hypotension, syncope, and shock. The reactions usually occur within minutes of taking aspirin and almost always occur within 1 h of ingestion. Patients may have cross-sensitivity to NSAIDs. Aspirin-induced asthma can be precipitated by NSAIDs but not usually by a nonacetylated salicylate salt, such as choline magnesium trisalicylate (Trilisate).

300. The answer is B. (*Wall, p 797.*) The acute syndrome associated with the administration of interferon, which occurs in almost all patients receiving the immunotherapy, consists of fever, chills, myalgias, arthralgias, and headache. Pretreatment with acetaminophen may decrease symptoms.

301. The answer is D. (*Wall, p 798.*) Patients receiving 20 to 100 mg dexamethasone intravenously should be warned that they may experience a transient burning sensation in the perineum. Administering the steroid slowly may prevent the perineal pain, the etiology of which is unknown.

302. The answer is D. (*Bonica, p 1678.*) The antidepressants with the greatest sedative effects are amitriptyline (Elavil), doxepin (Sinequan), trazodone (Desyrel), and maprotiline (Ludiomil). The least sedating antidepressants include imipramine (Tofranil), desipramine (Norpramin), amoxapine (Asendin), and protriptyline (Vivactil).

303. The answer is C. (*American Society of Regional Anesthesia [ASRA], p 283.*) General pharmacologic characteristics of antidepressants (tricyclics, tetracyclics, atypical and serotonin-specific reuptake inhibitors) include extensive absorption from the GI tract and extensive first-pass hepatic metabolism. They are highly bound to serum proteins (especially alpha-1 acid glycoprotein), are lipophilic, and have large volumes of distribution. Elimination half-lives are 1 to 4 days, and many have active metabolites.

304. The answer is D. (*Wall, p 428.*) Phenothiazines, lithium, cimetidine, and bumetanide (Bumex) can cause significant muscle cramping. Other conditions associated with muscle cramping are glycolytic disorders such as myophosphorylase deficiency (McArdle's disease) and phosphofructokinase (PFK) deficiency, dehydration, uremia, and hemodialysis. Benign, painful muscle cramping of unknown etiology can occur occasionally in healthy persons. Various symptomatic medical treatments have included use of quinine preparations, diazepam and other benzodiazepines, and muscle relaxants.

305. The answer is B. (*Bonica, p 1891.*) Epinephrine is combined with local anesthetics that have a short to moderate duration of action to prolong neural blockade. It causes a local vasoconstriction, which delays absorption of local anesthetic from the injection site and reduces systemic blood levels. The risk of systemic toxicity is thereby decreased. Use of epinephrine with lidocaine, procaine, or chlorprocaine prolongs neural blockade. Its use with bupivacaine or etidocaine does not significantly prolong neural blockade.

306. The answer is D. *(Bonica, p 1653.)* Constipation is the most frequent side effect of opioid therapy. Tolerance does not develop to this side effect. Therefore, as the dose of opioid increases, so does the potential for constipation. Frank bowel obstruction, biliary spasm, and ileus have occurred with opioid use. It is crucial to place patients on an active bowel regimen that includes laxatives, stool softeners, adequate fluids and exercise, and cathartics as needed to prevent the severe constipation that can occur with opioid use.

307. The answer is B. *(Bonica, p 1648.)* Morphine 10 mg IM is roughly equivalent to 120 mg codeine IM; 2 mg levorphanol IM; 100 mg meperidine IM; 10 mg methadone IM; and 2 mg hydromorphone (Dilaudid) IM. Oral morphine is one-third as potent as intramuscular or intravascular morphine. Therefore, 10 mg morphine IM is roughly equianalgesic to 30 mg orally.

308. The answer is D. *(Bonica, p 1677.)* The antidepressants appear to be analgesic independent of their effect on depression. They are thought to prevent reuptake of serotonin and norepinephrine in the descending antinociceptive pathways. Lower doses of antidepressants than those used for the treatment of depression have provided significant analgesia. The analgesic response usually occurs more rapidly than the antidepressive response (several weeks).

309. The answer is B. *(Brown, p 3.)* Tetracaine is a long-acting anesthetic used for spinal anesthesia and topical airway anesthesia. In spinal anesthesia, 1% tetracaine usually lasts 1.5 to 2.5 h. If epinephrine is added, it can last up to 4 h. It is not used for tissue infiltration. Procaine, lidocaine, and bupivacaine are all local anesthetics commonly used for tissue infiltration. Procaine without epinephrine lasts 1 h, and with epinephrine, up to 1.5 h. Lidocaine without epinephrine lasts 1 to 1.5 h, and with epinephrine up to 3 h. Bupivacaine lasts 3 to 6 h without epinephrine and is not significantly prolonged by the addition of epinephrine.

310. The answer is D. *(Brown, p 3.)* All local anesthetics have an aromatic end, an intermediate chain, and an amide end. They are subdivided into two groups: the ester and the amide local anesthetics. The amino esters have an amide linkage between the intermediate chain and the aromatic end. Esters include cocaine, procaine, 2-chloroprocaine, and tetracaine. Amides include lidocaine, mepivacaine, prilocaine, ropivacaine, bupivacaine, and etidocaine.

311. The answer is A. *(Wiener, p 221.)* Patients with acute acetaminophen overdose may present with a clinical picture that mimics viral hepatitis. A distinguishing characteristic is that with acetaminophen-induced hepatitis, the aspartate aminotransferase level often is ≥ 5000 U/L. Significantly lower levels are seen in viral hepatitis. Sodium acetylcysteine may protect the liver from lethal injury if given within 10 h of ingestion of a toxic dose of acetaminophen. Patients who suffer from chronic alcohol abuse have a very high risk of hepatotoxicity with even moderate doses of acetaminophen.

312. The answer is C. *(Wiener, p 252.)* This patient is manifesting signs of analgesic nephropathy. It is usually painless unless associated with renal papillary necrosis or infection. Chronic renal failure associated with daily use of 1 g or more of acetaminophen and aspirin for a period of more than 3 years describes analgesic abuse nephropathy. Hypertension, elevated creatinine, and anemia are common. Some or all of the renal failure will reverse itself if excessive analgesic use is discontinued.

313. The answer is D. *(Tollison, pp 185–188.)* Placebos are "therapeutic substances or procedures that are deliberately given to have an effect on a system, syndrome, or disease, but that are without specific activity for the condition being treated." Placebo has been shown, in some instances, to relieve pain in 35 percent of patients. The personality of the patient and cultural attitudes about pain play an important role in determining the degree of placebo response. The mechanism of response has been suggested to be psychological or behavioral, and even induction of the endogenous opioid system has been suggested. No mechanism has been definitely determined. Of note, peak effects, cumulative effect, and carry-over effects have been documented. Patients may report side effects similar to those seen with "active" drugs, such as nausea, headaches, thirst, dizziness, insomnia, depression, fatigue, numbness, difficulty concentrating, hallucinations, feelings of cold or warmth, and itching. Tolerance to placebo analgesia and an abstinence-like syndrome on cessation of placebo have occurred.

314. **The answer is E.** (*Wall, pp 938–939.*) Analgesic adjuvants enhance the response of known analgesics. Caffeine increases the analgesic effect and shortens time of onset of aspirin, acetaminophen, and ibuprofen. Amphetamines such as dextroamphetamine increase the analgesic effect of morphine sulfate and decrease its sedative effect. Hydroxyzine (an antihistamine) increases the analgesic effect of morphine and itself has some analgesic effect. It is mildly sedating as well. TCAs are useful adjuvant analgesics in cancer pain. Metoclopramide (Reglan) is not an analgesic adjuvant.

315. **The answer is D.** (*Tollison, pp 257–259.*) Preventive treatment of cluster headaches includes elimination of all alcohol, avoidance of daytime napping, and normalization of sleep cycle and daily activities. Prolonged sleeping should be avoided. Prednisone (3-week tapered regimen) is the most effective medication for control of cluster headaches. Lithium carbonate is also effective in 60 percent of cases. However, hypothyroidism may occur with long-term lithium use, and it may also be nephrotoxic. Use NSAIDs with caution in patients on lithium. Calcium-channel blockers may be very helpful. Methysergide and chlorpromazine have also been useful. NSAIDs may be effective, but appear to be most effective in the cluster headache variant called *chronic paroxysmal hemicrania*. In severe cluster headaches for which drug therapy has been ineffective, surgery and other ablative procedures of the sphenopalatine ganglion, cranial nerve V, and nervus intermedius have been effective in some cases.

316. **The answer is A.** (*Cousins, p 65.*) Vascularity and the presence of tissue and fat that can bind local anesthetics are primary influences on the rate of removal of local anesthetics from specific sites of injection. In general, independent of the specific agent used, the absorption rate decreases in the following order: intercostal block, caudal block, epidural block, brachial plexus block, sciatic and femoral nerve block.

317. **The answer is B.** (*Stoelting, p 2.*) Pharmacodynamics is the study of drug and receptor interaction. The major focus is on the chemical structure of the drug and the sensitivity of receptors to drugs. Pharmacokinetics describes the absorption, distribution, metabolism, and excretion of drugs in the body.

318. **The answer is D.** (*Stoelting, p 9.*) Most drugs will bind to some extent to the plasma proteins albumin, alpha-1 acid glycoprotein, and lipoproteins. Only the unbound portion is free and has pharmacologic activity at the receptors. Acidic drugs tend to bind primarily to albumin, and basic drugs bind to alpha-1 acid glycoproteins. If a drug is highly protein-bound, it remains in high plasma concentrations, with only small amounts passing into tissues. Therefore, the volume of distribution is small for a highly protein-bound drug.

319. **The answer is D.** (*Bonica, p 313.*) There is evidence that oral contraceptives, reserpine, propranolol, methyldopa, and prednisone in doses greater than 30 mg/day may induce or exacerbate existing depression. Opioids do not induce depression.

320. **The answer is D.** (*Bonica, p 317.*) Maprotiline has an increased risk of causing seizures. The occurrence can be minimized by starting at a low dose of 25 mg and increasing by 25 to 50 mg every 5 days until the daily dose of 150 mg is attained. Any further increment in dosing should be done slowly, using 25-mg increases over a 1-week period or more, closely monitoring the patient for side effects.

321. **The answer is B.** (*Bonica, p 317.*) Amoxapine is structurally related to loxapine, an antipsychotic drug. Akathisia is the most common extrapyramidal side effect of amoxapine, and if it develops, the drug should be discontinued and another antidepressant instituted. Patients manifesting the side effect of akathisia are likely to develop tardive dyskinesia with continued use of the drug.

322. **The answer is C.** (*Bonica, p 317.*) The given side effect profile is most characteristic of trazodone, a commonly used antidepressant. In medically healthy patients, the drug is very safe. Even large doses ingested in suicide attempts have failed to produce cardiotoxicity or fatality in patients without preexisting cardiac disease.

323. The answer is C. (*Bonica, p 1680.*) The patient is showing signs of mild withdrawal reactions, which can occur when tricyclic or tetracyclic antidepressants are discontinued without tapering. Symptoms of headache, diarrhea, and vivid dreams have occurred after abrupt discontinuation of even short-term use of low-dose heterocyclic antidepressants. To decrease the occurrence of the uncomfortable withdrawal symptoms, patients should taper off the medication slowly over a period of a few weeks.

324. The answer is C. (*Wall, p 888.*) Propranolol is a beta$_2$ antagonist that has been shown to enhance the analgesic effect of doxepin, a tricyclic antidepressant, in the treatment of central pain syndromes.

325. The answer is A. (*Robinson, JAMA 274:420–424, 1995.*) Strontium-89 is a pure beta-emitting radioisotope found to be effective in treatment of painful bony metastases. It has been most studied and most successfully used as palliative treatment in patients suffering from painful bony metastases from prostatic or breast cancer. It has a greater than 10-to-1 tumor-to-marrow absorbed dose ratio. Though it is relatively marrow-sparing in comparison with other isotopes (e.g., phosphorus-32), some degree of bone marrow suppression will occur. Strontium-89 is administered intravenously and pain relief occurs after 7 to 20 days if the therapy is successful.

326. The answer is D. (*Cheshire, Pain 59:65–69, 1994. Greene, Neurology 40:1213–1218, 1990.*) Relative contraindications to the use of botulinum toxin injections are myasthenia gravis and other muscle-weakening diseases and the use of aminoglycoside antibiotics. The aminoglycosides may potentiate the effects of the botulinum toxin or make its effect unpredictable. Use of tricyclic antidepressants is not a contraindication to use of botulinum toxin. The toxin has been used to effectively treat patients with strabismus, long-standing myofascial pain, and spasticity after spinal cord injury.

327. The answer is E. (*Cheshire, Pain 59:65–69, 1994. Greene, Neurology 40:1213–1218, 1990.*) The clinical effect of botulinum A toxin will be seen in 24 to 72 h after injection. The drug acts primarily in the periphery, at the neuromuscular junction, where it inhibits the release of acetylcholine. The toxin is produced by the bacterium *Clostridium botulinum*. The clinical effect may take several weeks to months to wear off, thereby offering prolonged relief to patients suffering from torticollis, strabismus, blepharospasm, and myofascial pain.

328. The answer is D. (*Ramamurthy, p 172.*) The amount of lithium excreted by the kidneys is sensitive to the sodium balance in the human body. With low sodium levels, there is less excretion of lithium, resulting in higher serum lithium concentrations. Careful attention should be paid to sodium balance to avoid marked changes in therapeutic level of the drug. Metabolism is not affected by sodium balance.

329. The answer is D. (*Bonica, p 531.*) Erythromelalgia is a condition in which a patient complains of severe burning pain associated with increased temperature of the skin due to abnormal vasodilation. The cause is unknown, though patients with hypertension, diabetes, lupus, rheumatoid arthritis, or venous insufficiency have a higher incidence of this rare disease. Treatment consists of having the patient avoid conditions (such as heat) that will increase vasodilation and exacerbate symptoms. Helpful medications include acetylsalicylic acid, phenoxybenzamine, and methysergide. Diphenylhydantoin has not been used in the treatment of erythromelalgia.

330. The answer is B. (*Ramamurthy, p 172.*) Tricyclic antidepressants (such as amitriptyline) inhibit the reuptake of serotonin and norepinephrine at nerve terminals. They also decrease the uptake of guanethidine (a long-acting alpha blocker) at nerve terminals, thereby decreasing its action as a potent vasodilator used in the treatment of reflex sympathetic dystrophy. The other substances listed do not affect the actions of guanethidine at the neural receptors.

331. The answer is C. (*Ramamurthy, p 176.*) The metabolism of prilocaine leads to the accumulation of the metabolite *ortho*-toluidine, which can convert hemoglobin to methemoglobin. When large doses of prilocaine are used, significant methemoglobinemia can occur. Treatment of methemoglobinemia is with intravenous methylene blue. The other local anesthetics listed do not have metabolites that can cause methemoglobinemia.

332. **The answer is B.** (*Fishbain, Clin J Pain 8:77–85, 1992.*) Drug and alcohol abuse, dependency, and addiction are not more common in patients with chronic pain. The prevalence of drug misuse in the chronic pain population is cited as 3.2 to 18.8 percent, which is not significantly higher than the prevalence in the general population. Careful monitoring is recommended when drugs with addictive potential are administered to any patients, with or without chronic pain.

333. **The answer is D.** (*Bonica, p 1684.*) Use of lithium is contraindicated in patients with renal tubular disease, myasthenia gravis, a history of myocardial infarction or cardiac conduction defects, and in early pregnancy. Lithium has been used to treat acute and chronic cluster headaches, painful shoulder syndrome, and pain associated with such psychological disorders as mania or recurrent depression.

334. **The answer is B.** (*Tollison, pp 63–67.*) Meperidine (Demerol) has a duration of action of 1 to 3 h. Butorphanol acts for 3 to 4 h, is an agonist-antagonist analgesic of the nalorphine type, is three to five times as potent as morphine and can only be given parenterally. Morphine has a duration of action of 3 to 5 h. MS-Contin is a slow-release, long-acting morphine preparation given two or three times a day.

335. **The answer is D.** (*Tollison, pp 479–480.*) Corticosteroids are potent anti-inflammatory agents, but do not have significant analgesic properties. They do not prevent progression of disease or destruction of joints. There is no evidence that one class of corticosteroids is more effective than another. Shorter-acting steroids are usually chosen because they have a low risk of suppression of the hypothalamic-pituitary-adrenal axis when used in appropriate dosages. Dexamethasone is the most potent and has the longest duration of action. Betamethasone is also long-acting. Triamcinolone is intermediate-acting. Hydrocortisone, prednisone, and methylprednisolone are short-acting. Prednisone and methylprednisolone are 4 times more potent than hydrocortisone. Triamcinolone is 5 times more potent than hydrocortisone. Betamethasone is 25 times and dexamethasone is 30 times more potent than hydrocortisone.

336. **The answer is B.** (*Tollison, p 553.*) The dose equivalents to 10 mg morphine are approximately 100 mg meperidine, 100 μg fentanyl, 500 μg alfentanil, and 10 mg methadone. Several physical and psychosocial factors may affect the actual dosage a patient may require to obtain analgesia. The pharmacokinetics of absorption can also be highly variable. Studies have shown that intrasubject variations in response to equianalgesic dosages of narcotics are small.

337. **The answer is D.** (*Savage, J Pain Symptom Management 8:265–278, 1993.*) Phenobarbital has been used successfully in the treatment of benzodiazepine withdrawal. The benzodiazepines are withdrawn slowly to minimize the physiologic effects. Morphine and tricyclic antidepressants are not commonly used to treat withdrawal syndromes. Diazepam, a long-acting benzodiazepine, has been used to treat alcohol withdrawal. Clonidine has been used to treat the symptoms of opioid withdrawal.

338. **The answer is C.** (*Gilman, pp 531–535.*) Symptoms of opioid withdrawal begin 8 to 12 h after the last dose. At this time, tearing, rhinorrhea, yawning, and sweating occur. By 12 to 24 h, the patient becomes restless, has dilated pupils, anorexia, gooseflesh, irritability, and tremor. Withdrawal symptoms peak at 48 to 72 h. The patient may complain of insomnia, severe sneezing, weakness, nausea and vomiting, intestinal cramps and diarrhea, abdominal pain, muscle cramps, and spasm. Tachycardia and hypertension, chills alternating with flushing, sweating, and piloerection occur. The patient should be closely monitored and treated for dehydration, ketosis, acidosis, leukocytosis and rare potential cardiovascular collapse. Seizures do not occur. Untreated withdrawal usually subsides in 7 to 10 days; withdrawal from long-acting opioids may be prolonged. The syndrome is rarely life-threatening.

339. **The answer is D.** (*Cousins, p 129.*) The amino esters (cocaine, procaine, chloroprocaine, tetracaine) are structurally related to paraaminobenzoic acid, which is a known allergen. Allergic reactions have occurred with the use of tetracaine. The amino amides include lidocaine, bupivacaine, mepivacaine, prilocaine, etidocaine, and ropivacaine. Allergic reaction to the amino amides is extremely rare, though there are a few documented reports.

PHARMACOLOGY ANSWERS

340. The answer is D. (*Campbell, APS Journal 1:3–11, 1992.*) Phentolamine is a short-acting, competitive, alpha-adrenergic antagonist that can be administered intravenously to aid in the diagnosis of sympathetically maintained pain, such as reflex sympathetic dystrophy. A few studies have suggested that it can predict patient response to intravenous regional guanethidine. It has been shown to be equally effective in relieving stimulus-independent and stimulus-evoked pain. The mechanism by which phentolamine exerts its effects is believed to be peripheral rather than central. There is no temperature rise expected to occur in the affected limb with infusion of intravenous phentolamine as there is with intravenous regional guanethidine or lumbar sympathetic block.

341. The answer is A (1,2,3). (*Raj, pp 608–612.*) The nonacetylated salicylates have less effect on platelet function and on gastrointestinal mucosa than the acetylated salicylates. However, the nonacetylated salicylates do produce similar degrees of analgesia and similar blood levels of salicylate to those of the acetylated salicylate drugs. Sulindac is a pyrrole acetic acid derivative that is chemically related to indomethacin.

342. The answer is B (1,3). (*Ferrante, p 165.*) With continued use of substantial amounts of opioid, the potency of the opioid declines so that progressively more and more drug is required to produce the same degree of analgesia. This phenomenon, called *tolerance*, is characteristic of opioids as a class of drugs. Tolerance can occur without physical dependence.

343. The answer is A (1,2,3). (*Ferrante, p 195.*) Naltrexone is an oral antagonist used in the treatment of opioid addictions. Cholecystokinin, nalorphine, and nalmefene are opioid antagonists, but are not used clinically. Naloxone is a parenteral antagonist used clinically to treat opioid overdose and respiratory depression. Given orally, it can decrease the ileus associated with opioid use.

344. The answer is E (all). (*Ferrante, p 186.*) The mixed agonist-antagonists (pentazocine, nalbuphine, butorphanol) and the partial agonists (and dezocine) exhibit all the listed properties. In addition, the antagonist properties may be used to reverse mu-agonist effects (respiratory depression, pruritus, nausea, and vomiting) while still preserving analgesia.

345. The answer is B (1,3). (*Ferrante, p 168.*) Histamine release is seen with the administration of morphine, codeine and meperidine. There is no histamine release associated with the administration of fentanyl, sufentanil, and oxymorphone.

346. The answer is C (2,4). (*Tollison, pp 254–256.*) Inhalation of 100% oxygen at 7 L/min for 15 min is effective in 75 percent of cluster headache patients. Use of ergotamine alkaloid can also abort attacks. Cyproheptadine and Bellergal are medications used to prevent migraines, not cluster headaches.

347. The answer is B (1,3). (*Ferrante, p 58.*) Clonidine (an alpha$_2$ agonist) inhibits discharge of nociceptive neurons in the dorsal horn and produces analgesia when applied to the spinal cord in animals and humans.

348. The answer is C (2,4). (*Cousins, p 41.*) Tachyphylaxis, a drug's declining effectiveness when it is given repeatedly, is often observed when a continuous nerve block is used over a long period of time. It is less likely to occur if a blocking agent is reinjected soon after the first signs of returning sensation. When the block is allowed to lapse, however, tachyphylaxis frequently occurs. Hallmarks of tachyphylaxis are ever shorter duration of action, fading anesthetic potency, and shrinking analgesic field. Chemical solutions that contain epinephrine and acidic antioxidants, such as sodium metabisulfate, increase the likelihood of tachyphylaxis.

349. The answer is C (2,4). (*Wall, p 429.*) Amphetamines, phencyclidine, alcohol, and diamorphine can cause a severe, acute rhabdomyolysis that is very painful. The subsequent myoglobinuria may precipitate renal failure. In addition, a polymyositis has been described in patients with Wilson's disease who are taking D-penicillamine. Muscle biopsies show muscle necrosis and an inflammatory reaction.

350. The answer is A (1,2,3). *(Stoelting, p 93.)* Buprenorphine is an agonist-antagonist opioid. Its analgesic potency is great: 0.3 mg IM is equivalent to 10 mg IM morphine. It is estimated that the affinity of buprenorphine for mu receptors is 50 times greater than that of morphine, and the lipid solubility is estimated to be at least 5 times that of morphine. About 96 percent of buprenorphine is bound to proteins, while only 30 to 35 percent of morphine is bound, primarily to albumin.

351. The answer is A (1,2,3). *(Raj, pp 375–380, 434–446. Tollison, pp 54–67.)* Addition of pentazocine, an agonist-antagonist analgesic, may precipitate withdrawal in patients taking opioid agonists. Once pathology requiring urgent treatment has been ruled out, the patient needs to have her medications adjusted to provide her with adequate analgesia. She has been taking MS-Contin 90 mg bid for 2 months and may have developed tolerance to this dose, or her metastases may have progressed. Therefore her dosing will need to be adjusted upward, while any side effects, such as constipation or nausea and vomiting, will need to be aggressively treated. Ibuprofen (an NSAID) in conjunction with opioids can provide excellent analgesia for bony metastases. The maximum recommended dose is 800 mg qid. The patient's renal function should be monitored. Evidence of easy bruising, gastritis, anemia, or CNS changes should be looked for in patients on chronic NSAIDs. TCAs have direct analgesic effects; they block reuptake of serotonin and norepinephrine at synapses in the descending pain-modulating network in the CNS.

352. The answer is B (1,3). *(Raj, p 615.)* Naproxen is a propionic acid derivative. It appears to be as effective an anti-inflammatory agent as aspirin, but is better tolerated. Naproxen is rapidly and extensively absorbed after both oral and rectal administration. Peak plasma concentrations routinely occur within 2 h after oral administration. Naproxen binds to plasma proteins extensively (99.6 percent). Its elimination half-life ranges from 12 to 15 h and is independent of the dose.

353. The answer is E (all). *(Ferrante, pp 280–283.)* When an opioid is delivered to the epidural space, all the listed actions occur. These characteristics affect the clinical effects of various opioids in the following way: Lipid-soluble agents (e.g., fentanyl) have rapid onset of analgesia, short duration, and early respiratory depression associated with the degree of systemic uptake. Hydrophilic agents (e.g., morphine) have slow onset of analgesia, prolonged duration, and late respiratory depression associated with rostral spread via the CSF to the brainstem.

354. The answer is A (1,2,3). *(Ferrante, pp 175, 187, 190, 191.)* *Butorphanol* is a mixed opioid agonist-antagonist. It acts as an antagonist at the mu receptor and an agonist at the kappa receptor (producing analgesia and sedation) and has low affinity for the sigma receptor. Therefore, it has a lower incidence of dysphoric reactions than pentazocine, which has higher sigma-receptor affinity. It can reverse pruritus caused by mu-agonist opioids. *Buprenorphine* is a partial mu-receptor agonist that has been used to reverse pruritus associated with epidurally administered mu agonists. *Nalbuphine,* a mixed agonist-antagonist, can be used to reverse respiratory depression and pruritus associated with mu agonists. It can also precipitate withdrawal symptoms in patients physically dependent on opioids. *Levorphanol* is a mu agonist that is most useful for treatment of chronic pain, most notably cancer pain.

355. The answer is B (1,3). *(Cousins, p 1058.)* The block produced by phenol tends to be less profound and of shorter duration than that produced by alcohol. Phenol has been used as a 5% to 6% solution in glycerine or as a 7.5% to 10% solution in iophendylate. Unlike absolute alcohol, phenol solutions are hyperbaric and viscous and deteriorate during storage. However, deterioration typically takes at least 1 year to occur.

356. The answer is E (all). *(Cousins, p 697.)* Convulsions are not the only complication of bolus injection into the internal carotid or vertebral artery. Total blindness, aphasia, hemiparesis, and unconsciousness of a transient and completely recoverable nature have also been reported.

357. The answer is B (1,3). (*Cousins, p 720.*) Intravascular injection should be avoided by aspirating repeatedly during injection of alcohol, phenol, or other neurolytic agents. Within a few seconds, intravascular injection of 10% phenol causes severe tinnitus and flushing, but recovery is rapid and complete. Accidental intravascular injection of absolute alcohol results in effects that are pleasurable and require no specific therapy. However, intravenous alcohol may sometimes cause thrombosis of the vessel.

358. The answer is A (1,2,3). (*Cousins, pp 224–225.*) The most important factors in determining the spread of spinal anesthetic solutions and the factors most susceptible to manipulation in order to achieve predictable levels of spinal anesthesia are the weight of the anesthetic solution injected in relation to the weight of CSF, the dosage and volume of anesthetic solution injected, and the position of the patient during and immediately after injection. Addition of a vasoconstrictor has no demonstrable effect on distribution of local anesthetic solution in the CSF.

359. The answer is B (1,3). (*Cousins, p 141.*) In multidose vials, methylparaben (1%) is often the antimicrobial included in local anesthetic solutions. Methylparaben is effective against gram-positive organisms and fungi but less so against gram-negative bacteria. It may be responsible for some of the allergic reactions attributed to local anesthetics.

360. The answer is A (1,2,3). (*Wall, p 796.*) Intrathecal methotrexate produces an acute meningitis in 5 to 50 percent of patients being treated for leukemia or leptomeningeal metastases. Intravenous L-asparaginase used to treat acute lymphoblastic leukemia can cause thrombosis of cerebral veins in 1 to 2 percent of patients. Transretinoic acid used in the treatment of acute myelocytic leukemia may cause hypervitaminosis. A pseudotumor cerebri may follow, causing a transient, severe headache. Intravenous 5-fluorouracil is associated with an increased incidence of ischemic chest pain, especially in patients with a prior history of coronary artery disease.

361. The answer is E (all). (*Wall, p 828.*) Tricyclic antidepressants with potent anticholinergic properties may increase the risk of anticholinergic delirium when taken in conjunction with other drugs with anticholinergic properties. Such other drugs include all those listed in the question.

362. The answer is B (1,3). (*PDR, 1995, pp 943, 2109, 2664.*) Fluoxetine and sertraline are SSRIs. Venlafaxine prevents the reuptake of both serotonin and norepinephrine, and to a lesser degree, dopamine. There is still some debate as to the analgesic efficacy of the SSRIs. The greatest analgesic efficacy has been demonstrated with antidepressants that block reuptake of both norepinephrine and serotonin.

363. The answer is E (all). (*Wall, p 834.*) It is important to remember that medications other than those the patient is receiving for pain may cause changes in mental status. Intrathecal methotrexate may cause delirium, dementia, lethargy, and personality changes. Vincristine and vinblastine may cause delirium, hallucinations, and lethargy. Bleomycin, carmustine (BCNU), 5-fluorouracil, and cisplatin can cause delirium.

364. The answer is C (2,4). (*PDR, 1995, p 1487.*) Patients who have used baclofen for prolonged periods should be withdrawn slowly from the medication. Abrupt withdrawal may precipitate seizures and hallucinations.

365. The answer is A (1,2,3). (*Raj, pp 76–77.*) The placebo effect is said to occur when an intervention that is not expected to have an effect produces one. In the case of analgesia it is clear that "sugar pills" are able to produce significant reductions in reported pain intensity in over 30 percent of the population. Pain cannot be measured directly. Likewise, the placebo effect cannot be measured accurately. The existence of this effect has made the double-blind crossover design the best study design to use in the evaluation of treatment modalities.

366. The answer is B (1,3). (*Raj, p 77.*) Just as interventions that are theoretically ineffective may produce beneficial effects, so may ineffective interventions produce adverse effects. Such negative placebo effects are also known as "nocebo" effects. These adverse effects are often the same as those expected from the active agent, especially when the subject has been fully informed of the potential adverse effects of the active agent. The occurrence of the nocebo effect during diagnostic or therapeutic maneuvers during pain management does not imply either presence or absence of nociceptive processes or of psychogenic pain. Currently, there are no psychological tests to predict the occurrence of nocebo effects.

367. **The answer is A (1,2,3).** (*Raj, p 845.*) There are several factors that seem to predispose patients to develop late-onset respiratory depression following spinally administered opioids. These include advanced age, large doses of opioids, use of water-soluble opioids, intrathecal opioids (versus the epidural route), concomitant use of parenteral opioids or sedatives, and thoracic epidurally administered opioids. Late-onset respiratory depression is also more likely in opioid-naive patients and high-risk patients.

368. **The answer is E (all).** (*Raj, p 594.*) Volumes of distribution are apparent volumes describing the dilution of the total amount of drug within the body. Distribution is an interaction between a drug and the body. It is affected by such physiologic properties of the body as local pH, tissue composition, permeability of membranes, and blood flow.

369. **The answer is A (1,2,3).** (*Tollison, pp 254–256.*) Medications used to prevent recurrence of migraine include beta blockers, methysergide, calcium-channel blockers, antidepressants, NSAIDs, cyproheptadine, clonidine, Bellergal, and occasionally dilantin, tegretol, or baclofen. Cyproheptadine can be used alone and is the treatment of choice for prevention of childhood migraines. Methysergide (Sansert) should not be used for more than 6 months at a time because of the risk of retroperitoneal fibrosis as well as fibrosis of the lungs and heart valves. Intravenous pyelography, chest radiography, and cardiac examination should be performed after 6 months of taking methysergide, or earlier if symptoms develop. The fibrosis may be reversible in some cases. Lithium is used as a preventive treatment for cluster headaches, but not migraine headaches.

370. **The answer is E (all).** (*Tollison, pp 252–254. Wall, p 500.*) Drugs used to treat acute migraine attacks include ergotamine tartrate and dihydroergotamine. Ergotamine is mainly an arterial vasoconstrictor, but it may also have a central effect. Ergotamine preparations can be administered via intravenous, intramuscular, subcutaneous, oral, rectal, inhalational, or sublingual routes. The drug should not be used in patients with hypertension, peripheral vascular disease, coronary artery disease, collagen vascular disease, or thrombophlebitis or in patients over age 60. It can cause GI upset and bradycardia. Use with extreme caution in patients on beta blockers.

Isometheptene is a sympathomimetic and is found in combination with acetaminophen and dichloralphenazone, a mild tranquilizer. The combination drug is called Midrin. It causes fewer GI symptoms than ergotamine and is useful in mild to moderate attacks.

NSAIDs such as naproxen sodium, meclofenamate sodium, indomethacin, and ibuprofen may be helpful as symptomatic and as preventative medications.

Sumatriptan is primarily a 5-HT-D agonist. It is a rapid, highly effective intramuscular medication that can abort migraine attacks. Use cautiously in patients with hypertension and coronary artery disease.

Other medications used to treat migraine symptoms include narcotics; phenothiazines, which are effective antiemetics and may also have some pain-relieving benefit (chlorpromazine, promethazine, hydroxyzine); and metoclopramide.

371. **The answer is E (all).** (*Raj, p 594.*) Volumes of distribution are affected by physiologic properties of the body and physiochemical properties of the drug. Physiochemical properties of the drug include degree of ionization, lipid solubility, polarity, and molecular weight.

372. **The answer is C (2,4).** (*Cousins, p 129.*) Reports of allergic reactions to local anesthetic agents appear periodically. Unfortunately, systemic toxic reactions to local anesthetic agents are frequently misdiagnosed as representing allergic or hypersensitivity-type reactions. The amino-ester agents that are derivatives of para-aminobenzoic acid (PABA), a known allergen in nature, have been shown to produce allergic-type reac-

tions. Reactions of an allergic type to the amino-amide agents, which are not derivatives of PABA, are extremely rare but have occurred. Multidose containers of amino-amide agents may contain the preservative methylparaben, whose chemical structure is similar to PABA.

373. **The answer is A (1,2,3).** (*Ferrante, pp 311, 312, 317.*) Tachyphylaxis is the development of acute tolerance to the effect of epidural local anesthesia. A given dose of local anesthesia becomes less effective with repeated dosing. Tachyphylaxis has occurred in patients who were receiving either intermittent injections or continuous infusions epidurally. Lower concentrations of local anesthetics seem to be associated with a lower incidence of tachyphylaxis than higher concentrations. Tachyphylaxis is best documented in patients receiving bupivacaine or lidocaine. Adding epinephrine to lidocaine seems to decrease the incidence of tachyphylaxis. Coadministration of intravenous or epidural opioids restores the efficacy of epidural local anesthetic and may prevent further development of tachyphylaxis.

374. **The answer is E (all).** (*Bonica, pp 1982–1983.*) The primary effect of phenol is to coagulate protein. Like alcohol, there is nonselective damage to nervous system tissue. The degree and extent of the lesion is dependent upon the volume and concentration used. Phenol has a transient local anesthetic effect and is therefore less painful than alcohol on injection. Phenol in glycerin is hyperbaric to CSF on injection, but rapidly decreases to isobaricity in 15 min. This suggests that it is probably safe for patients to change position at that time, though it is frequently recommended that position should be maintained for 45 min.

375. **The answer is B (1,3).** (*Bonica, p 1983.*) A solution of 50% glycerol has been used to successfully treat trigeminal neuralgia without producing significant sensory loss. Injection into the trigeminal ganglion is more damaging than topical application. There is extensive myelin disintegration, axonolysis, and wallerian degeneration, which continues to occur weeks after injection.

376. **The answer is E (all).** (*Braga, Agents Actions 41:121–131, 1994.*) Calcitonin is a polypeptide hormone found to have a significant analgesic action. It has been used to provide significant pain relief to patients with such varied conditions as phantom limb pain, Paget's disease, osteoporosis, metastatic bone lesions, vertebral compression fractures, rheumatoid arthritis, Tietze's syndrome, fibromyalgia, and reflex sympathetic dystrophy. It is usually administered intranasally or intramuscularly. It can also be administered epidurally or intrathecally, though there is a higher incidence of nausea and vomiting associated with these routes.

377. **The answer is E (all).** (*Cheshire, Pain 59:65–69, 1994. Greene, Neurology 40:1213–1218, 1990.*) Botulinum toxin A has been used to treat strabismus, myofascial pain, blepharospasm, and torticollis with significant improvement in pain symptoms. The effect can last up to several months, though it may be 1 to 3 days before the clinical effect can be seen after injection.

378. **The answer is E (all).** (*Raj, p 555.*) Patients suffering from a painful sensory neuropathy associated with AIDS often complain of burning dysesthesias of the feet, which can be disabling as well as painful. Treatment with tricyclic antidepressants, carbamazepine, phenytoin, topical capsaicin, and opioids in combination with low-dose amitriptyline has been helpful in alleviating the symptoms associated with AIDS neuropathy.

379. **The answer is B (1,3).** (*Bonica, p 1654.*) Addiction describes the psychological dependence on the use of a particular drug associated with craving of the drug for effects other than pain relief. The addicted person's attention is constantly focused on obtaining and using the drug. There is a high incidence of relapse after withdrawal. Withdrawal symptoms occur in persons who have developed a physical dependence on a drug. If there is no psychological dependence (addiction), the relapse rate is very low. Hospitalized patients and cancer patients have an extremely low incidence of addiction.

380. **The answer is A (1,2,3).** (*Ramamurthy, p 172.*) Hepatic enzyme-inducing drugs or states that increase hepatic blood flow will increase the clearance of other drugs. Phenytoin, barbiturates, and smoking may increase induction of hepatic enzymes. Propranolol and cimetidine may lower the clearance of such drugs as local anesthetics and benzodiazepines.

381. The answer is E (all). (*Tollison, p 479.*) Osteoporosis, avascular necrosis of bone, hypertension, glucose intolerance, and cataract formation are major risks associated with the chronic use of corticosteroids. Though corticosteroids are commonly used in the treatment of chronic joint and connective tissue pain, their use remains controversial. However, there is general consensus that corticosteroid therapy is appropriate in the treatment of systemic lupus erythematosus.

382. The answer is B (1,3). (*Gilman, pp 522–573.*) Clonidine, an alpha-adrenergic agonist, and buprenorphine, a mixed agonist-antagonist opioid, have been used to successfully treat the symptoms of opioid withdrawal. Hydroxyzine, dicyclomine, and triazolam may be helpful as well. Clonidine should be administered around the clock in a tapered protocol over the first 7 days of withdrawal. Buprenorphine is given in a tapered regimen every 4 h over the first 6 days of withdrawal. After discontinuation of the medication, the patient is observed for continued symptoms of withdrawal before detoxification is considered complete. It is extremely important for the patient to have the psychological and social supports in place before discharge in order to decrease the risk of relapse.

383. The answer is B (1,3). (*Savage, J Pain Symptom Management 8:265–278, 1993.*) Long-acting benzodiazepines are the most commonly administered medications to prevent the onset of potentially lethal delirium tremens during abstinence from alcohol. Dosages should be high enough to prevent symptoms of delirium tremens and should be tapered slowly as the patient undergoes detoxification in a setting that provides psychological and social support to the recovering alcoholic. Lorazepam and diazepam are long-acting benzodiazepines. Clonidine and buprenorphine have been used in opioid detoxification programs.

384. The answer is C (2,4). (*Ramamurthy, p 172.*) Alkalinizing the urine by use of sodium bicarbonate or acetazolamide results in increased reabsorption of tricyclic antidepressants, thereby decreasing the rate of excretion and drug clearance. There is no effect on drug metabolism, which occurs in the liver.

Medical and Surgical Techniques of Pain Management

DIRECTIONS: Each question below contains suggested responses. Select the **one best** response.

385. All the following statements regarding superior laryngeal nerve block are true EXCEPT that

    (A) the block is performed at the inferior border of the hyoid bone
    (B) it can produce motor blockade of the cricoarytenoid muscles
    (C) the local anesthetic is deposited deep to the thyrohyoid membrane
    (D) the superior laryngeal nerve is a branch of the vagus nerve
    (E) anesthesia results over the inferior aspect of the epiglottis

386. When performing a "third occipital nerve block," it is important to know that this nerve is a branch of the dorsal rami of

    (A) C1
    (B) C2
    (C) C3
    (D) C4
    (E) C5

387. Landmarks used in performing a cave of Retzius block include the

    (A) costophrenic angle
    (B) anterior superior iliac spine
    (C) L2 vertebral body
    (D) os pubis

388. A splanchnic nerve block is correctly characterized by which statement?

    (A) It is performed at the L1 level
    (B) It is performed with the needle at the posterolateral aspect of the vertebral body
    (C) It is recommended for surgical anesthesia
    (D) It requires a larger volume of local anesthetic than celiac plexus block
    (E) It can result in a chylothorax

389. When performing an inguinal perivascular block, one should

    (A) insert the needle just medial to the femoral artery
    (B) inject a volume of 10 to 15 mL of local anesthetic
    (C) hold pressure proximal to the needle insertion site
    (D) search for a paresthesia

390. Advantages of the interscalene approach to blocking the brachial plexus include all the following EXCEPT that

    (A) it can be performed with the arm in any position
    (B) it can also block the cervical plexus
    (C) there is less risk of pneumothorax
    (D) a low volume of solution is required

391. The block in the figure below would be most indicated for

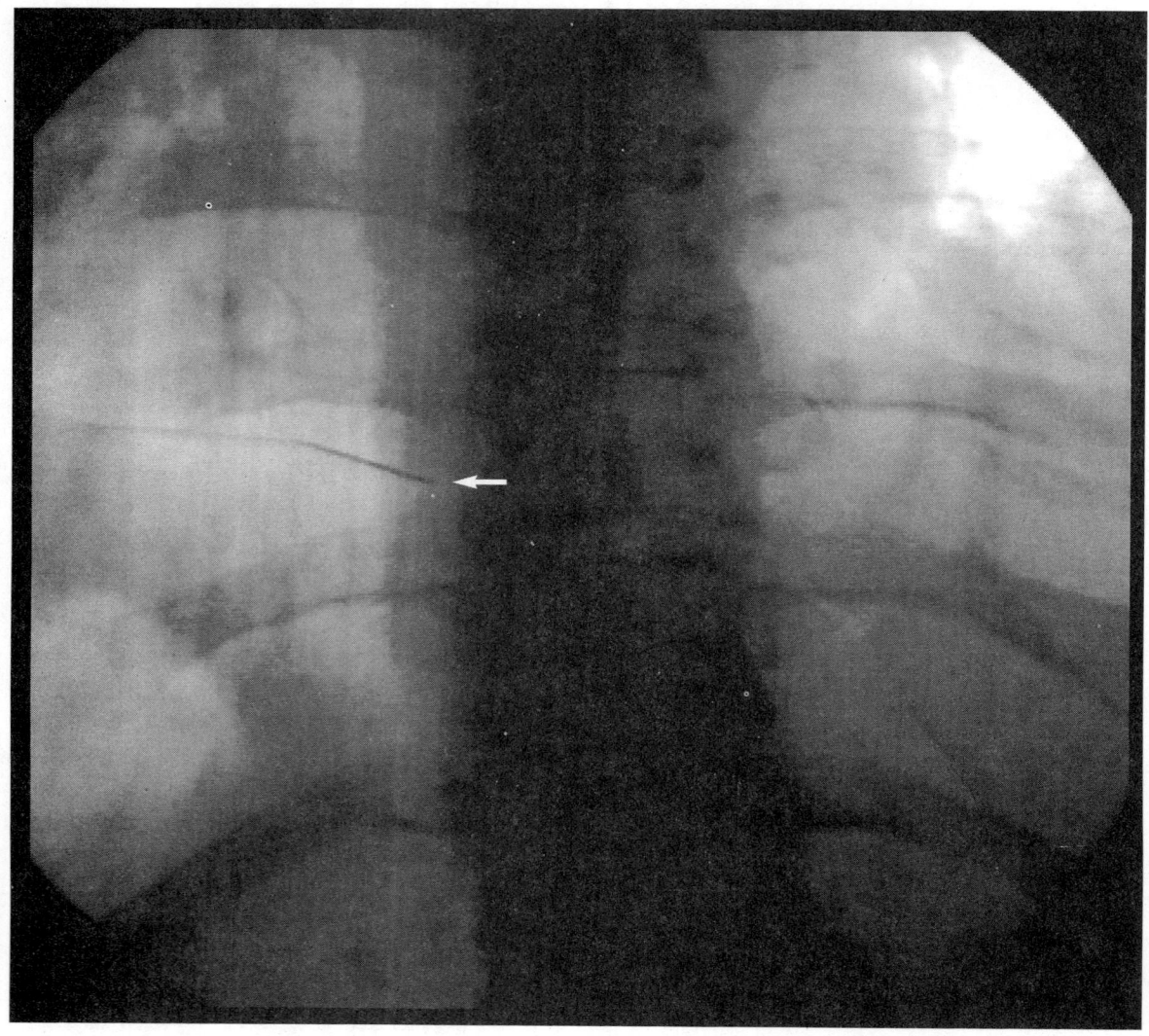

- (A) pleuritic pain
- (B) sympathetically maintained pain
- (C) acute herpes zoster
- (D) postherpetic neuralgia
- (E) chronic pancreatitis

392. The figure below illustrates

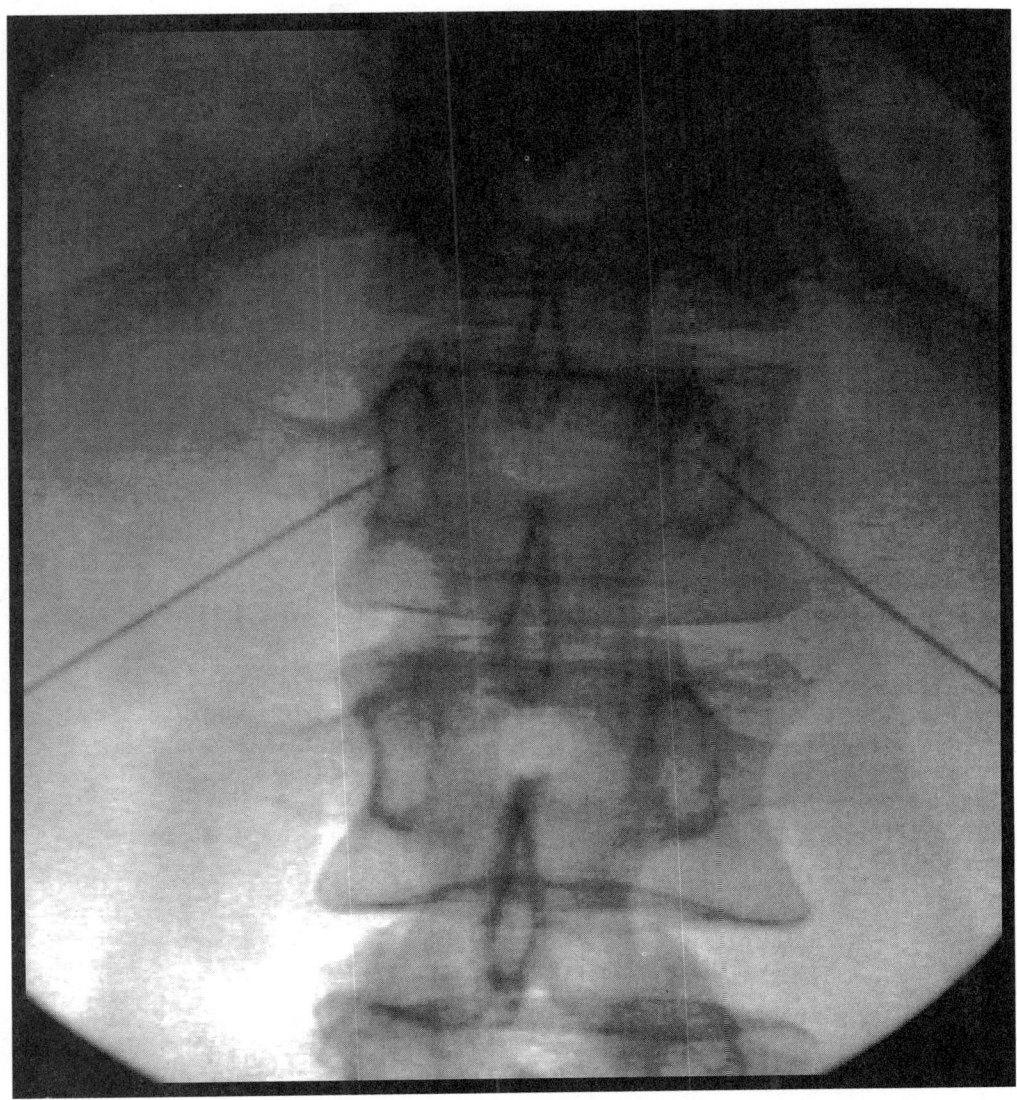

(A) splanchnic nerve block
(B) superior hypogastric plexus block
(C) lumbar sympathetic block
(D) celiac plexus block
(E) bilateral somatic nerve block

393. The block in the figure below would be most helpful for a patient suffering from

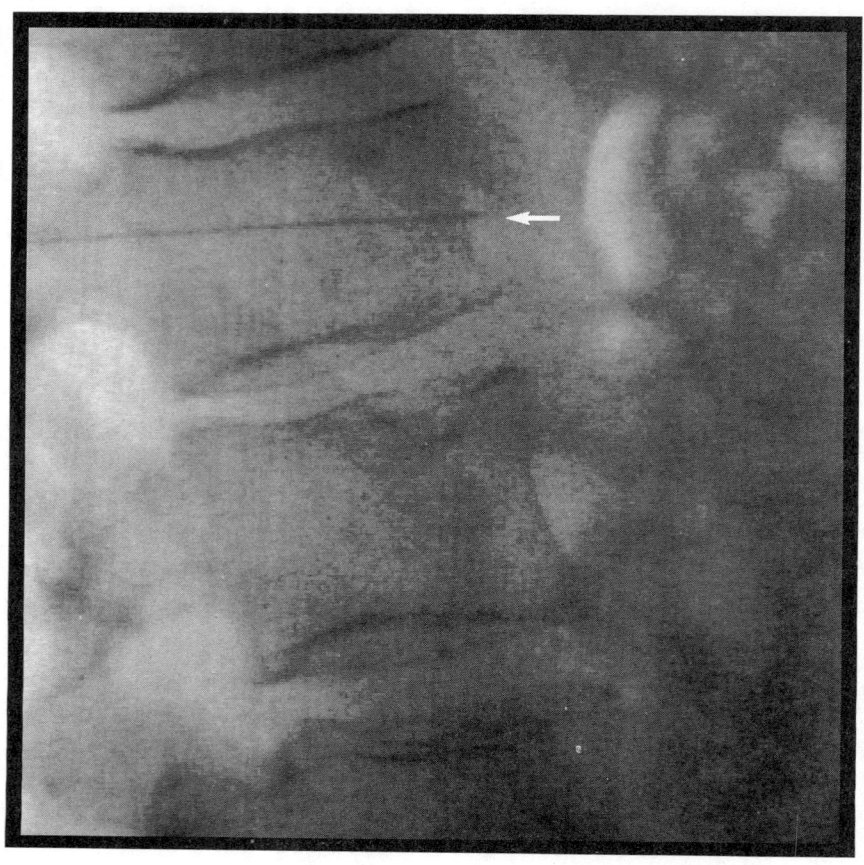

- (A) acute lumbar herniated disk
- (B) neuropathic pain in the foot
- (C) lumbar facet joint arthropathy
- (D) acute lumbar strain
- (E) sympathetically maintained pain in the leg

394. The spinal needle with a "pencil point" is also known as the

(A) Touhy needle
(B) Quincke-Babcock needle
(C) Greene needle
(D) Pitkin needle
(E) Whitacre needle

395. The Taylor approach for performing a lumbar puncture is commonly performed at which interspace?

(A) L1–L2
(B) L2–L3
(C) L3–L4
(D) L4–L5
(E) L5–S1

396. Treatment of steroid pseudorheumatism should consist of

(A) benzodiazepines
(B) rest
(C) steroids
(D) NSAIDs

397. A celiac plexus block is very helpful in relieving pain from each of the following EXCEPT

(A) hepatic cancer
(B) gastric cancer
(C) uterine cancer
(D) cholangiocarcinoma
(E) pancreatic cancer

398. A 21-year-old man is complaining of left groin and thigh pain 2 days after undergoing a left-sided neurolytic lumbar sympathetic block for reflex sympathetic dystrophy of the left leg. The most likely diagnosis is

(A) persistent reflex sympathetic dystrophy
(B) lumbar plexopathy
(C) lumbar radiculopathy
(D) genitofemoral neuralgia
(E) meralgia paresthetica

399. Which agent destroys nerves by producing wallerian degeneration (axonal degeneration without disruption of the Schwann cells)?

(A) Alcohol
(B) Methotrexate
(C) 5% Lidocaine
(D) Propylene glycol

400. The most common complication seen after a retrobulbar injection is

(A) perforation of the globe
(B) optic nerve damage
(C) intravascular injection
(D) retrobulbar hemorrhage
(E) oculocardiac reflex

401. All the following statements regarding the treatment of the pain associated with multiple sclerosis (MS) are true EXCEPT

(A) carbamazepine is the treatment of choice for MS-associated trigeminal neuralgia or paroxysmal extremity pains
(B) antidepressants have been recommended as treatment of nonparoxysmal extremity pain associated with MS
(C) dorsal column stimulation is a highly successful and recommended treatment for MS-associated extremity pain
(D) intrathecal baclofen has been used to successfully treat pain associated with severe spasticity

402. A 27-year-old woman with a history of malignant melanoma and multiple subcutaneous metastases has been successfully managed with slowly increasing doses of MS-Contin, in conjunction with doxepin and ibuprofen. She calls the pain center to complain of a new onset of increasing nausea, vomiting, and headaches, as well as poor pain control. The most appropriate immediate action would be to

(A) speak with the patient by telephone and tell her to increase the MS-Contin
(B) schedule the patient for an evaluation in your office within the week
(C) add ondansetron for nausea and vomiting so she is able to continue to take oral analgesics
(D) switch to a fentanyl patch since the patient is nauseated and may be unable to take oral analgesics
(E) see the patient as soon as possible to determine if there is a new, treatable source of pain

403. The most effective initial treatment for trigeminal neuralgia is

(A) baclofen
(B) tocainide
(C) phenytoin
(D) oxycodone
(E) carbamazepine

404. TENS has been shown to be effective in all the following clinical settings EXCEPT

(A) after thoracotomy
(B) diabetic neuropathy
(C) labor
(D) after upper abdominal surgery
(E) chronic low back pain

405. Contraindications to therapeutic heat include all the following EXCEPT

(A) chronic tendinitis or bursitis
(B) acute inflammation
(C) fresh hematoma
(D) pressure sores
(E) sensory loss

406. The physiologic effects of cold that are considered beneficial include all the following EXCEPT

(A) decreased metabolic rate
(B) decreased muscle spasm
(C) decreased nerve conduction velocity
(D) decreased spontaneous neural discharge
(E) decreased collagen distensibility

407. Which of the following statements is true regarding isometric exercise?

(A) The joint moves through its normal range
(B) It is the exercise of choice in patients with hypertension
(C) It requires expensive equipment to perform effectively
(D) It may be useful in a patient whose entire leg is in a cast
(E) It is not beneficial to patients with acute inflammatory arthritis

408. Traction has been used in the treatment of neck and low back disorders. All the statements about traction below are true EXCEPT

(A) in cervical traction, the angle of pull is 20 to 25° forward flexion with maximum weight of 22 kg
(B) to successfully perform lumbar traction, a pulling force of 40 kg or more may be needed
(C) traction is believed to enlarge intervertebral foramina, separate facet joints, and stretch muscles and ligaments
(D) it is safe to use in patients with osteoporosis, osteomyelitis, and rheumatoid arthritis
(E) active peptic ulcer and hiatal hernia are relative contraindications to lumbar traction

409. All the following complications of acupuncture can occur EXCEPT

(A) fainting
(B) pneumothorax
(C) needle breakage
(D) infection
(E) massive hemorrhage

410. The physiologic effects of massage are claimed to include all the following EXCEPT

    (A) improved perfusion of soft tissue
    (B) production of soft tissue edema and induration
    (C) rapid elimination of waste products
    (D) loosening and stretching of contracted tissues
    (E) production of relaxation and a sense of well-being

411. The conditions for which spinal manipulation is most frequently suggested include all the following EXCEPT

    (A) low back pain, especially if associated with degenerative changes of the facet joints
    (B) chronic headaches of unknown etiology when full work-up is negative
    (C) coccygodynia
    (D) chronic cervical pain, usually in the presence of degenerative disk disease
    (E) realignment of spine after vertebral fracture

412. A 16-year-old boy sustained a traumatic amputation of the left leg and subsequently developed phantom limb pain. All conservative therapies have been unsuccessful. The patient is scheduled for a trial of spinal cord stimulation. At what level should the electrodes be placed?

    (A) Middle to lower thoracic region
    (B) Upper to middle thoracic region
    (C) Lumbar region
    (D) Middle to lower cervical region

413. All the following have been successfully treated with spinal cord stimulation EXCEPT

    (A) failed back surgery syndrome
    (B) cancer pain
    (C) postamputation pain
    (D) reflex sympathetic dystrophy

414. The best results will be obtained from spinal cord stimulation when

    (A) unipolar electrodes are used
    (B) electrodes are localized at the dermatomal level of the pain
    (C) electrodes are placed intrathecally
    (D) the patient has no secondary gain from the pain

415. A gastroenterologist has referred a patient to you with abdominal pain and the diagnosis of biliary dyskinesia. The patient had increased basal sphincter pressure on biliary manometry and delayed biliary emptying. An endoscopic sphincterotomy was performed. However, the pain was relieved only a slight degree. The patient is told to expect "some blocks" to be performed. Which prognostic block would be most appropriate?

    (A) Celiac plexus block
    (B) Splanchnic block
    (C) Intercostal nerve block
    (D) Impar ganglion block

416. Which of the following statements is true regarding management of burn pain?

    (A) Narcotics remain the drugs of choice for treatment of acute, severe burn pain
    (B) Tolerance does not develop with the use of ketamine for burn therapy over an extended period of time
    (C) Silver sulfadiazine cream (Silvadene) is a potent topical anesthetic
    (D) Biofeedback has not been shown to be effective in reducing anxiety and pain in children with severe burns

417. You are consulted by a medical intern for evaluation and treatment of painful leg ulcers on a 76-year-old man. You note 2 × 3 cm ulcers on the medial malleoli. The surrounding tissue is hyperpigmented and indurated. There is bilateral pitting edema of the ankles. What treatments would you suggest for this patient?

    (A) Tylenol with codeine and prednisone
    (B) Elevation of the legs and support stockings
    (C) Capsaicin cream and antibiotics
    (D) Surgical excision of the ulcer and indurated tissue with primary closure

418. All the following statements regarding patient-controlled analgesia (PCA) pumps are true EXCEPT

(A) all PCA pumps have data storage capabilities
(B) a key and code numbers are required to make any changes
(C) a demand bolus can be administered while a baseline continuous infusion is running
(D) the number of times the button may be pushed during a dosing interval is limited

419. A 56-year-old man has an interpleural catheter in his left chest for pain relief from multiple rib fractures. He has a continuous infusion of 0.25% bupivacaine running at 6 mL/h but is still complaining of pain. On physical examination you notice that his left pupil is miotic. However, he is hemodynamically stable. The next logical step would be to

(A) stop the infusion
(B) increase the infusion rate
(C) order an emergent neurologic examination
(D) bolus the catheter
(E) change solution to 0.5% bupivacaine

420. A 64-year-old man has a lumbar epidural catheter in place for postoperative pain control after undergoing a low anterior resection. On physical examination, the patient is unable to flex his hips, extend his knees, and dorsiflex his right ankle. He would be assessed a Bromage score of

(A) 2
(B) 3
(C) 5
(D) 7
(E) 10

421. While performing a brachial plexus block with the aid of a nerve stimulator, you notice the onset of pronation of the arm, flexion of the wrist, and opposition of the thumb and forefinger. Which of the following nerves is most likely being stimulated?

(A) Ulnar
(B) Median
(C) Radial
(D) Musculocutaneous
(E) Brachioradialis

422. All the following complications have occurred after dorsal column stimulation EXCEPT

(A) infection at the incision site
(B) persistent incisional tenderness
(C) dislocation of the stimulating electrode
(D) bleeding and infection in the epidural space
(E) accelerated rate of epidural tumor growth

423. In the performance of a lumbar sympathetic block, injection of 15 to 20 mL of local anesthetic at the anterior aspect of the vertebral bodies of L2 or L3 will interrupt the sympathetic innervation of which of the following structures?

(A) Kidney
(B) Adrenal gland
(C) Ureter
(D) Prostate
(E) Ascending colon

424. In a selective posterior rhizotomy,

(A) a 1- to 2-mm incision is made in the ventrolateral aspect of the rootlet-cord junction
(B) no anesthesia is required
(C) the rootlet is completely divided
(D) only one rootlet at each level may be incised
(E) pial vessels may be safely incised

425. A 75-year-old man with unilateral thoracic wall pain secondary to multiple rib metastases is scheduled to undergo intrathecal phenol neurolysis. Which of the following statements is true regarding intrathecal phenol neurolysis?

(A) The patient should be positioned with the painful side up
(B) Phenol is painful on injection
(C) Phenol acts immediately on contact with the dorsal root
(D) A 25-gauge spinal needle should be used to inject the phenol
(E) After injection of phenol brings the desired effect, the patient's position should be maintained for 45 min

426. When performing an intrathecal neurolytic block of the left C7 to T1 nerve roots using absolute alcohol, which of the following positions would be most appropriate?

(A) Left side up
(B) Left side down
(C) Sitting
(D) Prone
(E) Supine

427. A patient with intractable cancer pain is scheduled to undergo percutaneous C1–C2 cordotomy on the left. This can be expected to provide analgesia in which part of the body?

(A) Left thorax, abdomen, leg, and hand
(B) Below the waist on the left side
(C) Below the waist on the right side
(D) The entire right side below the clavicle including the leg and the inner aspect of the right arm, right forearm, and hand
(E) The entire left side beginning below the mandible and including the left arm, thorax, abdomen, and leg

428. Treatment of priapism may include all the following EXCEPT

(A) spinal or caudal anesthesia
(B) aspiration of the corpus cavernosa
(C) surgical shunt of blood from the corpus cavernosa to the saphenous vein
(D) vitamin E and steroid injections
(E) narcotic pain relief and sedation

DIRECTIONS: Each question below contains four suggested responses of which **one or more** is correct. Select

A	if	**1, 2, and 3**	are correct
B	if	**1 and 3**	are correct
C	if	**2 and 4**	are correct
D	if	**4**	is correct
E	if	**1, 2, 3, and 4**	are correct

429. The joint in the figure below is

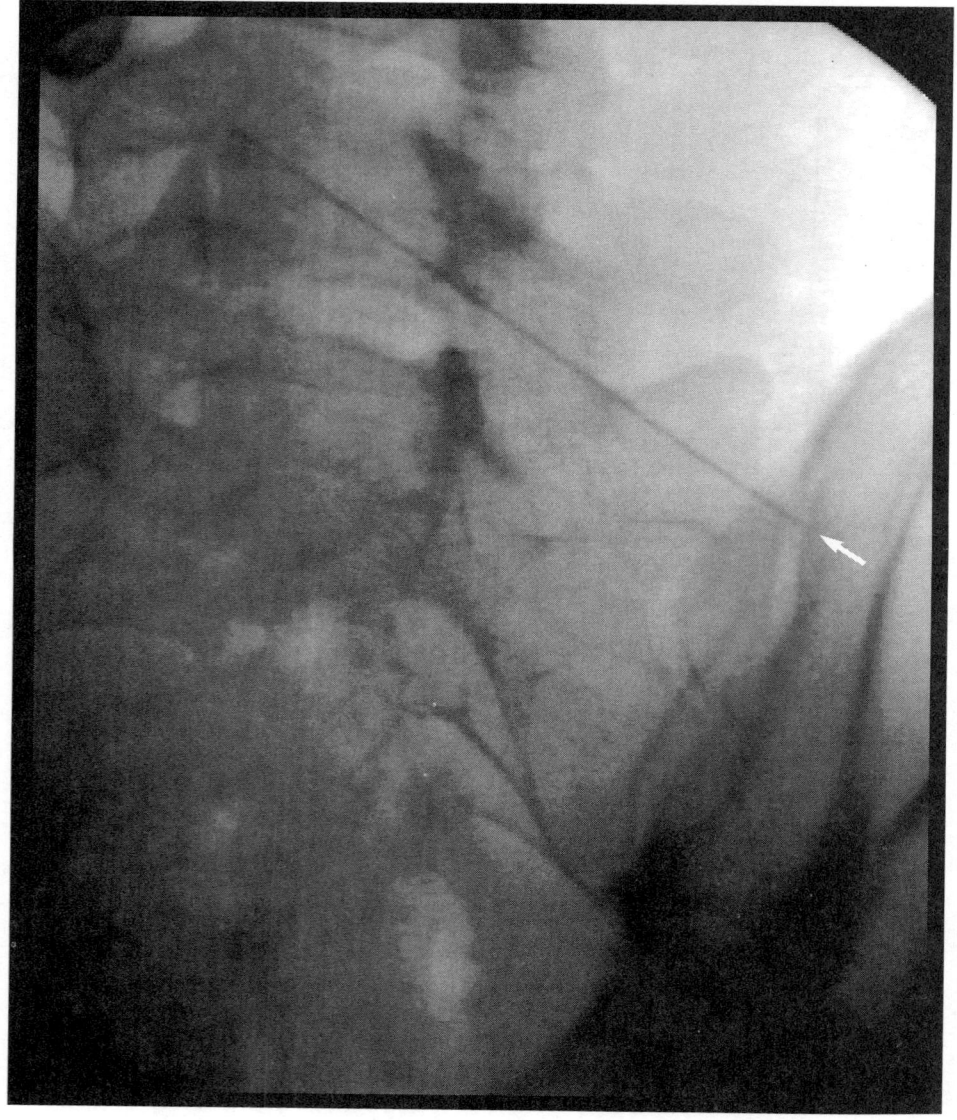

(1) a true joint consisting of two irregular articulations
(2) most susceptible to injury when lifting
(3) weakest anteriorly
(4) relatively unstable

430. The figure below illustrates the site for

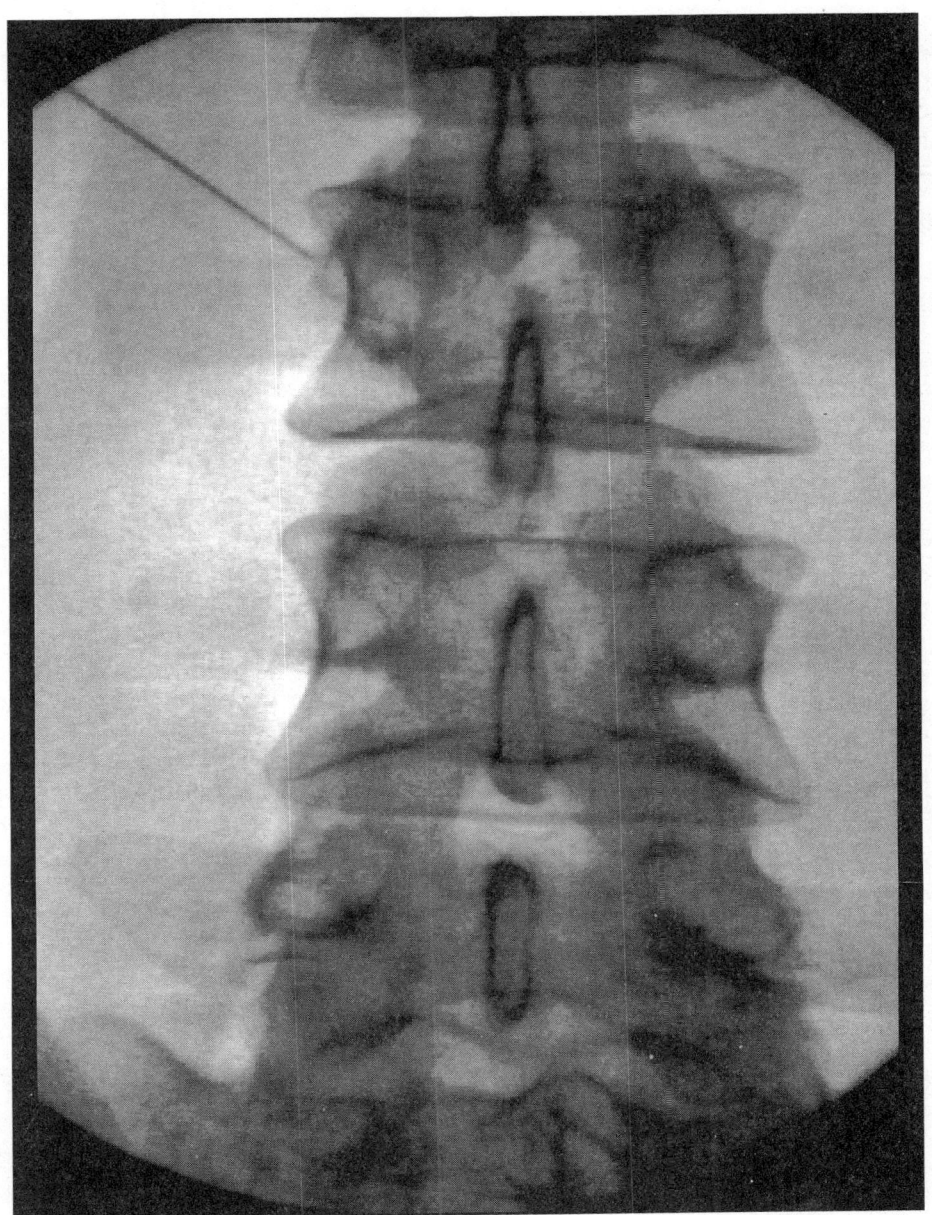

(1) medial branch block
(2) selective nerve root block
(3) facet joint denervation
(4) pars interarticularis injection

SUMMARY OF DIRECTIONS				
A	B	C	D	E
1,2,3 only	1,3 only	2,4 only	4 only	All are correct

431. Indications for dorsal root entry zone (DREZ) lesioning include

    (1) brachial plexus avulsion
    (2) postparaplegic or postquadriplegic pain
    (3) postamputation pain
    (4) postherpetic neuralgia

432. True statements regarding cryolesioning include

    (1) it is associated with less fibrous tissue reaction than other forms of destruction
    (2) it completely disrupts the endoneurium
    (3) it causes wallerian degeneration with axonal disintegration
    (4) it uses nitric oxide as the refrigerant gas

433. When performing an intrathecal alcohol block for pain in the chest wall, the

    (1) volume of injectate should be small
    (2) patient should be placed in an oblique lateral position
    (3) rate of injection should be slow
    (4) patient should be placed with the affected side down

434. Epidural steroid injections can

    (1) alter blood glucose levels in susceptible patients
    (2) cause a rash
    (3) cause fluid retention
    (4) depress plasma cortisol levels for 4 to 6 weeks

435. True statements regarding lumbar medial branch block include

    (1) a facet joint can be completely anesthetized by blocking one medial branch
    (2) medial branches arise from dorsal rami
    (3) each median nerve crosses the lower border of the lower transverse process
    (4) each medial branch enters the multifidus muscle

436. Intercostal nerve block is highly effective in relieving severe pain resulting from

    (1) costochondral dislocation
    (2) rectus nerve entrapment
    (3) acute herpes zoster
    (4) pleurisy

437. Local anesthetic nerve blocks may be helpful in which of the following neuropathic pain syndromes?

    (1) Trigeminal neuralgia
    (2) Diabetic neuropathy
    (3) Lumbosacral plexalgias
    (4) Entrapment syndrome

438. Which of the following can occur after neurolytic celiac plexus block?

    (1) Unilateral leg paralysis
    (2) Loss of function of the bladder sphincter
    (3) Hypotension
    (4) Decreased bowel motility

439. When performing an intravenous regional Bier block, which of the following is likely to result in high venous pressure with resultant systematic administration of solution?

    (1) Rapid injection
    (2) Injection into a distal vein
    (3) Large volume of injectate
    (4) Prolonged exsanguination

440. True statements regarding the ilioinguinal nerve include that it

    (1) lies superficial to the fascia of the external oblique muscle
    (2) originates from the T12 and L1 spinal levels
    (3) does not pass through the inguinal canal
    (4) is blocked near the anterior superior iliac spine

441. Characteristics of the common peroneal nerve include that it

    (1) originates at the apex of the popliteal fossa
    (2) is typically blocked at the neck of the fibula
    (3) lies medial to the biceps femoris muscle
    (4) lies superficial to the popliteal fascia

442. Blockade of the deep cervical plexus is aided by locating the

 (1) C6 transverse process
 (2) cricoid cartilage
 (3) mastoid process
 (4) ramus of the mandible

443. For complete anesthesia of the mandible, which of the following must be blocked?

 (1) Lingual nerve
 (2) Long buccal nerve
 (3) Inferior alveolar nerve
 (4) Masseter nerve

444. Infiltration of local anesthetic at the midpoint of the posterior border of the sternocleidomastoid will block the

 (1) lesser occipital nerve
 (2) greater auricular nerve
 (3) anterior cervical nerve
 (4) supraclavicular nerve

445. Blockade of the greater occipital nerve is aided by locating the

 (1) mastoid process
 (2) superior nuchal line
 (3) external occipital protuberance
 (4) temporal artery

446. An accessory nerve block is

 (1) performed superficial to the prevertebral fascia
 (2) used as an adjunct for shoulder surgery under regional anesthesia
 (3) performed at the junction of the middle and superior thirds of the sternocleidomastoid muscle
 (4) accomplished in the anterior triangle of the neck

447. Possible sequelae of a glossopharyngeal nerve block include

 (1) ipsilateral sternocleidomastoid muscle weakness
 (2) ipsilateral trapezius muscle weakness
 (3) tracheal numbness
 (4) hoarseness

448. Important landmarks used when performing a glossopharyngeal nerve block include

 (1) styloid process
 (2) angle of the mandible
 (3) mastoid process
 (4) zygomatic arch

449. True statements regarding a glossopharyngeal nerve block include that it commonly

 (1) results in blockade of CN X
 (2) results in blockade of CN XII
 (3) results in blockade of CN XI
 (4) is performed just below the foramen ovale

450. In the performance of a maxillary nerve block by a lateral approach, which of the following anatomic structures may be entered?

 (1) Infratemporal fossa
 (2) Parotid gland
 (3) Maxillary artery
 (4) Pterygopalatine fossa

451. In the performance of a combined infratrochlear and anterior ethmoidal nerve block, the needle should be

 (1) inserted 1 cm above the inner canthus
 (2) inserted to a depth of 4 cm
 (3) inserted on the medial wall of the orbit
 (4) directed posteriorly and slightly laterally

452. Nerves that lie in the same vertical plane as the pupil in midposition include

 (1) supraorbital
 (2) mental
 (3) infraorbital
 (4) supratrochlear

453. Landmarks used for performing an interscalene block of the brachial plexus include

 (1) anterior scalene muscle
 (2) cricoid cartilage
 (3) external jugular vein
 (4) sternocleidomastoid muscle

SUMMARY OF DIRECTIONS				
A	B	C	D	E
1,2,3 only	1,3 only	2,4 only	4 only	All are correct

454. A successful obturator nerve block is demonstrated by

    (1) Abductor paresis
    (2) Adductor paresis
    (3) Numbness over the anterior aspect of the thigh
    (4) Numbness over the medial aspect of the thigh

455. A lateral femoral cutaneous nerve block can be performed

    (1) 2 cm inferior and medial to the anterior superior iliac spine
    (2) after contacting the iliac bone just medial to and below the anterior superior iliac spine
    (3) deep to the fascia lata
    (4) deep to the external oblique aponeurosis

456. In the performance of a sciatic nerve block, the classic approach of Labat involves

    (1) positioning the patient lying on the side opposite the one to be blocked
    (2) placing the lower extremities in an extended position
    (3) drawing a line that coincides with the upper border of the piriformis muscle
    (4) drawing a trisected line over the inguinal ligament

457. With the standard techniques for performing a transsacral block, which of the following complications can occur?

    (1) Intravascular injection
    (2) Parasympathetic block
    (3) Subarachnoid injection
    (4) Sympathetic block

458. Landmarks commonly used in a transsacral block include

    (1) posterior superior iliac spine
    (2) iliac crest
    (3) sacral cornu
    (4) posterior inferior iliac spine

459. The lumbar plexus lies between which muscles?

    (1) Quadratus lumborum
    (2) Iliacus
    (3) Psoas
    (4) Piriformis

460. Complete sensory anesthesia of the thumb may involve which of the following blocks?

    (1) Radial nerve
    (2) Median nerve
    (3) "Ring"
    (4) Lateral cutaneous nerve of the forearm

461. The musculocutaneous nerve can be blocked

    (1) in the substance of the coracobrachialis muscle
    (2) lateral to the biceps tendon at the intercondylar line
    (3) 5 cm proximal to the intercondylar line
    (4) medial to the brachial artery at the intercondylar line

462. Important landmarks for a radial nerve block at the wrist include which of the following tendons?

    (1) Flexor carpi radialis
    (2) Extensor pollicis longus
    (3) Palmaris longus
    (4) Extensor pollicis brevis

463. Radial nerve block at the elbow uses which of the following anatomic landmarks?

    (1) Lateral epicondyle
    (2) Intercondylar line
    (3) Biceps tendon
    (4) Brachial artery

464. Landmarks commonly used in an ulnar nerve block at the wrist include

    (1) flexor carpi ulnaris
    (2) palmaris longus
    (3) ulnar artery
    (4) flexor retinaculum

465. Other nerves that can be blocked as a result of an interscalene plexus block include

    (1) inferior cervical ganglia
    (2) vagus nerve
    (3) phrenic nerve
    (4) recurrent laryngeal nerve

466. Possible complications of a supraclavicular brachial plexus block include

    (1) neuritis
    (2) block of phrenic nerve
    (3) toxic reaction
    (4) Horner's syndrome

467. True statements regarding the development of a pneumothorax after a supraclavicular brachial plexus block include

    (1) it is less likely to occur with finer needles
    (2) the occurrence rate is approximately 15 percent
    (3) the majority of cases take up to 24 h to develop
    (4) it is more common in obese patients

468. Factors affecting the spread of local anesthetic after injection in the caudal canal of adults include

    (1) speed of injection
    (2) age of patient
    (3) dose
    (4) height of patient

469. Bony landmarks commonly used for a caudal block include

    (1) posterior inferior iliac spine
    (2) sacral cornua
    (3) sacral crest
    (4) posterior superior iliac spine

470. Advantages of the supraclavicular approach to performing a brachial plexus block include

    (1) it blocks the plexus at the level of the trunks
    (2) a low volume of solution is required
    (3) there is quick onset time to block
    (4) all the plexus is reliably blocked

471. Landmarks commonly used when performing a supraclavicular brachial plexus block include the

    (1) sternocleidomastoid muscle
    (2) external jugular vein
    (3) subclavian artery
    (4) lateral third of the clavicle

472. Chemical hypophysectomy for pain relief in patients with cancer

    (1) is less successful than surgical hypophysectomy
    (2) is more successful than transnasal cryoprobe ablation
    (3) relieves pain in less than half of these patients
    (4) usually provides rapid pain relief

473. Electrocardiographic findings indicative of lidocaine toxicity include

    (1) increased PR interval
    (2) sinus bradycardia
    (3) increased QRS duration
    (4) complete atrioventricular (AV) dissociation

474. Opioid-induced pruritus has been successfully treated with

    (1) naloxone
    (2) naltrexone
    (3) nalbuphine
    (4) hydroxyzine

475. Interpleural analgesia can provide relief of pain from

    (1) mastectomy
    (2) nephrectomy
    (3) cholecystectomy
    (4) pancreatic cancer

476. Signs that occur in the presence of Horner's syndrome include

    (1) ptosis
    (2) myosis
    (3) enophthalmos
    (4) anhidrosis

SUMMARY OF DIRECTIONS

A	B	C	D	E
1,2,3 only	1,3 only	2,4 only	4 only	All are correct

477. When using a nerve stimulator to perform a peripheral nerve block,

    (1) motor response should be obtained with close to 1 milliampere (mA) of current
    (2) accuracy is increased if a coated needle is used
    (3) the anode of the stimulator should be attached to the needle
    (4) a motor response should be obtained at only minimal current output

478. Negative pressure in the lumbar epidural space increases

    (1) if a blunt needle with side openings is used
    (2) as the needle advances across the epidural space toward the dura
    (3) if the needle is introduced slowly
    (4) in the sitting position

479. True statements regarding epidural neurolysis include that

    (1) it is indicated for thoracic and upper abdominal wall pain
    (2) baricity of the injectate must be considered
    (3) it can be carried out over 2 to 3 days
    (4) positioning of the patient is of paramount importance

480. Clinical symptoms suggestive of a subdural block with local anesthetic include

    (1) widespread sensory or motor blockade
    (2) unilateral block
    (3) a delay in time before onset of symptoms
    (4) involvement of cranial nerves

481. Retrobulbar injection of local anesthetic provides akinesia of the extraocular muscles by blocking which of the following cranial nerves?

    (1) VI
    (2) III
    (3) IV
    (4) VII

482. Therapeutic modalities that may be effective in neuropathic pain include

    (1) neural blockade
    (2) neurosurgical interruption
    (3) narcotics
    (4) anti-inflammatory agents

483. Therapeutic modalities that may be useful in treating intractable chronic pain include

    (1) anti-inflammatory agents
    (2) neural blockade
    (3) narcotics
    (4) antidepressants

484. Characteristics of a sympathetic nerve block include that

    (1) it is considered successful if a rise in temperature occurs in the affected area
    (2) it may provide pain relief secondary to increased blood flow
    (3) it can be achieved by blocking a somatic nerve
    (4) it interrupts only afferent sympathetic activity

485. Treatment of coccygodynia may include

    (1) neurolytic nerve blocks
    (2) caudal cryoanalgesia
    (3) caudal epidural steroid injections
    (4) sacral rhizotomy

486. Treatment for central poststroke pain syndrome may include which of the following?

    (1) TENS
    (2) Antiepileptic drugs
    (3) Antidepressants
    (4) Peripheral neurolysis

487. Relative contraindications to the use of TENS include

(1) implanted cardiac pacemaker
(2) pregnancy
(3) dementia
(4) cephalic application in an epileptic

488. Deep brain stimulation can be used to treat

(1) facial anesthesia dolorosa
(2) thalamic syndrome
(3) postcordotomy dysesthesia
(4) chronic abdominal and perineal pain

489. Spinal cord stimulation (SCS) has been used to treat which of the following painful syndromes?

(1) Postamputation neuralgia
(2) Reflex sympathetic dystrophy (RSD)
(3) Phantom limb pain
(4) Ischemic pain

490. The most frequent indications for cold laser therapy include

(1) reduction of pain associated with acute trauma of tendons and ligaments
(2) acceleration of wound healing and reduction of edema
(3) reduction of chronic pain associated with osteoarthritis or rheumatoid arthritis
(4) peripheral nerve regeneration immediately following injury

491. The term *iontophoresis* refers to the

(1) use of direct current to cause muscle contraction in a denervated state
(2) use of an electrical current to induce chemical changes on the skin
(3) use of alternating current to stimulate innervated muscles
(4) transfer of ions across a tissue plane

492. Superficial heating modalities include

(1) hydrocollator pack
(2) ultrasound
(3) paraffin wax
(4) short-wave diathermy

493. A 66-year-old woman presents with known cervical facet arthropathy at the C5–C6 facet joint. She is to undergo cryoneurolysis in an attempt to provide pain relief. Cryoneurolysis should be performed at

(1) C4–C5
(2) C6–C7
(3) C5–C6
(4) C3–C4

494. Important principles of acute pain therapy include

(1) establishing drug levels to maintain analgesia
(2) reevaluating therapy regularly to meet the needs of individual patients
(3) determining the source and degree of nociception
(4) providing therapy for nociception and other components of suffering such as anxiety

495. Landmarks for performing a median nerve block at the elbow include the

(1) brachial artery
(2) lateral epicondyle
(3) medial epicondyle
(4) biceps tendon

496. Cryolesioning produces its analgesic effects by causing

(1) wallerian degeneration
(2) disruption of the myelin sheath
(3) axonal disintegration
(4) disruption of the Schwann cell basal lamina

497. When performing a celiac plexus block, which of the following are important external landmarks?

(1) 12th ribs
(2) T12 spinous process
(3) L1 spinous process
(4) L2 spinous process

SUMMARY OF DIRECTIONS				
A	B	C	D	E
1,2,3 only	1,3 only	2,4 only	4 only	All are correct

498. True statements regarding hypnosis as an adjunctive technique for the treatment of pain include which of the following?

   (1) The greater the level of hypnotic susceptibility, the greater the likelihood of pain reduction
   (2) It has been shown to be very effective in the treatment of painful burns
   (3) Both sensory pain and the suffering components of acute pain are reduced
   (4) The reduction of pain is most likely due to a placebo effect

499. True statements regarding lumbar epidural analgesia with lidocaine include which of the following?

   (1) Blockade below T6 in healthy, normovolemic patients does not produce significant decreases in blood pressure
   (2) Blockade to T3 decreases cardiac output
   (3) In hypovolemic patients, blockade to T4 will cause significant decreases in heart rate, cardiac output, and mean arterial pressure
   (4) Blockade of T3–T12 does not decrease mean arterial pressure in normovolemic patients

500. In a stellate ganglion block, injection of 15 mL of local anesthetic solution will spread sufficiently to involve the sympathetic innervation of which of the following structures?

   (1) Esophagus
   (2) Head and neck
   (3) Lungs
   (4) Stomach

501. When performing a celiac-splanchnic block, injection of 15 to 25 mL of local anesthetic solution bilaterally will spread sufficiently to block the sympathetic innervation of which of the following structures?

   (1) Descending colon
   (2) Pancreas
   (3) Rectum
   (4) Liver and gallbladder

502. True statements regarding treatment of osteoarthritis include

   (1) regular use of salicylates and NSAIDS will slow the progression of the disease
   (2) intraarticular corticosteroid injections every 2 weeks are useful as adjunctive therapy to oral medications
   (3) there is very high patient compliance with outpatient physical therapy
   (4) weight reduction for obese patients and assistive devices can help decrease pain

503. Contraindications to spinal column manipulation include which of the following?

   (1) Cervical osteophytes
   (2) Fixed posterior lumbar facet syndrome
   (3) Cervical degenerative joint disease with reduced disk height
   (4) Spondylolisthesis

504. Blockade of the hypogastric plexus will relieve pain caused by which of the following structures?

   (1) Uterus
   (2) Ovaries
   (3) Testes
   (4) Transverse colon

505. For which of the following painful conditions is circumcision a recommended treatment?

   (1) Phimosis
   (2) Balanitis
   (3) Paraphimosis
   (4) Condyloma acuminata

Medical and Surgical Techniques of Pain Management

Answers

385. **The answer is B.** (*Cousins, p 548.*) The superior laryngeal nerve is a branch of the vagus nerve and is easily blocked as it sweeps around the inferior border of the greater cornu of the hyoid bone. As the needle is "walked off" the inferior border of the hyoid bone, local anesthetic is injected both superficially and deep to the thyrohyoid membrane. This will produce anesthesia over the inferior aspect of the epiglottis and the laryngeal inlet as far down as the vocal cords.

386. **The answer is C.** (*Cousins, p 940.*) The C3 dorsal ramus forms two medial branches: a deep medial branch and a superficial medial branch known as the third occipital nerve. The deep medial branch follows a course around the C3 articular pillar and innervates the C3–C4 zygapophysial facet joint from above. The superficial medial branch, or third occipital nerve, pierces the splenius capitis and trapezius muscles just medial to the greater occipital nerve. It travels in the scalp fascia up to the vertex of the skull.

387. **The answer is D.** (*Cousins, pp 527–528.*) The variable space located between the urinary bladder and symphysis pubis is known as the cave of Retzius. This space contains a great venous plexus, as well as many terminating nerve fibers of the sacral plexus. Typically, a 7- to 8-cm needle is directed to the posterior aspect of the os pubis and anterior to the bladder. Ten milliliters of local anesthetic solution is injected as the needle reaches its maximum depth and is slowly withdrawn. The process is repeated with two lateral injections made through the same skin wheal.

388. **The answer is E.** (*Cousins, pp 521–522.*) The splanchnic nerves can be blocked above the diaphragm, at the upper border of T12, using techniques similar to a celiac plexus block. However, the needle is directed to the anterolateral angle of the vertebral body of T12. This block is not recommended for surgical anesthesia. For diagnosis and treatment of chronic abdominal pain, it is possible to obtain pain relief with a much smaller volume of solution than is the case with celiac plexus block. Complications include pneumothorax, vascular puncture, and thoracic duct damage, which may lead to a chylothorax.

389. **The answer is D.** (*Cousins, p 420.*) The technique for inguinal perivascular block is very similar to that for femoral nerve block. The needle is inserted just lateral to the femoral artery, where it emerges distal to the inguinal ligament. A paresthesia of the femoral nerve must be produced as an indication that the tip of the needle is within the fascial sheath. A volume of 25 to 30 mL of local anesthetic should be injected while digital pressure is applied just distal to the needle in an attempt to force the flow of local anesthetic proximally.

390. **The answer is D.** (*Cousins, p 398.*) Interscalene block is suitable when a proximal block is required, such as for shoulder surgery, when it is often necessary to block the cervical plexus. In addition it can be performed with the arm in any position. The risk of pneumothorax is reduced. It is essential to elicit paresthesias while performing this block, and unless large volumes are used, lower trunk anesthesia may be missed.

391. The answer is C. (*Raj, p 531.*) Since nerve root involvement is suspected in acute herpes zoster, somatic nerve blocks have been used in its treatment. These blocks can include brachial plexus, paravertebral, intercostal, and sciatic blocks. Such blocks have been found to be of some value in the acute phase and of no value in the postherpetic stage of herpes zoster infection.

392. The answer is D. (*Raj, pp 795–798.*) The celiac plexus lies anterior to the aorta and epigastrium. When performing this block, helpful landmarks include the spinous processes of T12 and L1 and the inferior border of the 12th rib. Classically, the needles are advanced to contact the lateral borders of the body of the L1 vertebra, then redirected and advanced to lie just anterior (2 to 3 cm) to the lateral part of the L1 vertebral body.

393. The answer is E. (*Raj, p 803.*) The lumbar sympathetic chain lies at the anterolateral border of the vertebral bodies. Lumbar sympathetic blocks have been used extensively in the treatment of reflex sympathetic dystrophy and causalgia. Most fibers headed for the lower extremity pass through the second and third lumbar ganglia so that a sympathetic block placed at this level will provide almost complete sympathetic denervation to the lower extremity.

394. The answer is E. (*Cousins, p 238.*) The Quincke-Babcock spinal needle has a sharp point with a medium-length cutting bevel. The Pitkin spinal needle has a sharp point but short bevel, with cutting edges and a rounded heel. The Greene spinal needle has a rounded point and a rounded, noncutting bevel of medium length. The Whitacre spinal needle, or the "pencil point needle," has a completely rounded, noncutting bevel with a solid tip. The opening of the needle is on the side, 2 mm proximal to the tip of the needle.

395. The answer is E. (*Cousins, p 242.*) The Taylor approach is a special paramedian approach to enter the L5 interspace (between L5 and S1), the largest interlaminar space. The patient is placed in a flexed lateral decubitus position and a spinal needle is inserted 1 cm medial and 1 cm caudad to the lowest part of the posterior-superior iliac spine. The needle is directed medially and cephalad to an angle of 55° into the subarachnoid space.

396. The answer is C. (*Wall, p 796.*) The treatment for steroid pseudorheumatism is to administer steroids and taper the drug very slowly.

397. The answer is C. (*Raj, p 795.*) Any pain originating from visceral structures and innervated by the celiac plexus can be effectively alleviated by blockade of the celiac plexus. This includes the pancreas, liver, gallbladder, omentum, mesentery, and alimentary tract from the stomach to the transverse colon. Pain from uterine cancer is more likely to respond to a superior hypogastric plexus block rather than celiac plexus block.

398. The answer is D. (*Raj, p 808.*) The genitofemoral nerve is most susceptible at the L4–L5 vertebral level, after it has emerged from the psoas major muscle and lies anterior to the fascia in close proximity to the sympathetic chain. Lateral spread of neurolytic solution from the lumbar sympathetic chain can result in genitofemoral neuralgia and, less often, involvement of the lumbar plexus.

399. The answer is A. (*Raj, pp 707–709.*) At 50 to 100%, alcohol causes wallerian degeneration of axons without destroying the Schwann cell tube. Axonal regeneration will usually occur over time. At 3 to 12%, phenol will also cause axonal degeneration, and recovery of function is usually faster than with alcohol. Other neurolytic agents include 50% glycerol, 10% ammonium chloride, chlorocresol, and the aminoglycoside streptomycin.

400. The answer is D. (*Cousins, p 588.*) Retrobulbar hemorrhage is the most common complication seen after a retrobulbar block. It is characterized by increasing proptosis and subconjuctival blood. An oculocardiac reflex may occur some hours after a retrobulbar hemorrhage as additional blood extravasates. Following a recognized retrobulbar hemorrhage, surgery should be postponed until all signs of hemorrhage have resolved, usually within 2 to 4 days.

401. The answer is C. (*Wall, p 895.*) Treatment of MS-related pain consists of antiepileptic drugs (AEDs) for patients with trigeminal neuralgia or paroxysmal extremity pains. Carbamazepine is a first-line drug, though other AEDs have also been used successfully. Antidepressants are recommended as treatment for the burning, nonparoxysmal pain associated with MS with varying success. TENS may be tried. However, dorsal column stimulation has had poor results and is not recommended as treatment for MS-related pain. Severe spasticity may cause pain in patients with MS. This has been successfully treated with intrathecal baclofen.

402. The answer is E. (*Jacox, p 38.*) Changes in pain patterns or the development of new pain should be evaluated thoroughly. New pain may be due to fracture, infection, or progression of the disease to a new area. A change in the quality or intensity of the pain may be due to advancing disease. In this case, the patient had new metastases to the area postrema, which caused intractable nausea as well as further progression of her disease to multiple, deep sites.

403. The answer is E. (*Wall, pp 705–706.*) Approximately 70 percent of patients with trigeminal neuralgia will get significant relief from carbamazepine (Tegretol). Phenytoin (Dilantin) is an effective drug to be used if carbamazepine is not helpful. Baclofen has also been used with some success, though side effects are frequent. Tocainide has efficacy similar to that of carbamazepine. However, it is not used because of the potential for lethal side effects. Oxycodone and other narcotic analgesics may be used acutely, but they are not helpful in the long-term management of recurrent trigeminal neuralgia.

404. The answer is C. (*Ferrante, pp 457–473. Raj, pp 673–675.*) TENS involves a gating mechanism in the dorsal horn of the spinal cord, where large-diameter, myelinated A fibers that mediate light touch and pressure interact with the small-diameter, unmyelinated C fibers that transmit pain sensation. Both A and C fibers synapse onto interneurons of the substantia gelatinosa (laminae II and III) that send impulses to the cells in lamina V. If C-fiber input predominates, presynaptic inhibition is decreased and painful stimuli ascend to the somatosensory cortex. If stimulation of A fibers predominates (they are more easily stimulated), presynaptic inhibition of laminae II and III cells occurs and transmission of pain impulses is blocked. Two types of TENS commonly used are those of high frequency (80 to 100 Hz) with low intensity (50 to 80 μs) and acupuncture-like stimulation of low frequency (10 Hz) with high intensity (200 μs). Biphasic waveforms with amplitude set by the patient to comfortable tingling are usually well tolerated. Onset of analgesia for high-frequency, low-intensity stimulation is immediate; it may not be reversed by naloxone, but may be reversed by serotonin. Onset of analgesia for low-frequency, high-intensity stimulation is 20 to 30 min and may be reversed by naloxone. This form of TENS may be especially helpful in chronic pain. TENS is used to treat acute postoperative pain, chronic low back pain, arthritis, phantom limb pain, reflex sympathetic dystrophy, and peripheral neuropathies.

405. The answer is A. (*Tollison, pp 148–150.*) Heat therapy is used for symptomatic pain relief and relaxation in chronic pain patients. Patients usually undergo treatment for 20 min at temperatures below 45°C (113°F). At temperatures higher than 45°C, warmth is no longer the primary sensation and pain occurs. Commonly used superficial heating devices include hot water bottles, heating pads, hydrocollator packs, paraffin wax, and heat lamps. Deep heating devices include short-wave diathermy, microwave diathermy, and ultrasound. Contraindications to heat therapy include its use on anyone who cannot respond to impending burn (babies, mentally confused, patients with sensory loss) and its use on ischemic areas or pressure sores, acutely inflamed areas, recent hematomas, or tumors. Short-wave and microwave diathermy should not be used in patients with cardiac pacemakers or patients with metallic implants in the area being treated. Ultrasound should not be used over fluid-containing organs such as the eyes or gravid uterus. It is safe to use over metallic implants since bone and metal are equally dense to ultrasound.

406. The answer is E. (*Tollison, pp 150–151.*) Beneficial effects of cold include (1) decreased metabolic rate with decreased inflammation; (2) decreased muscle spasm because cold muscle does not contract effectively; (3) decreased nerve conduction velocity and spontaneous neural discharges; and (4) analgesia via the gate mechanism. Physiologic effects of cold that may not augment analgesia are the joint stiffness that occurs as synovial fluid viscosity increases and the decrease in collagen distensibility, which may make stretching exercises less effective.

407. The answer is D. (*Tollison, p 152.*) Isometric exercises are muscle strengthening exercises in which there is *no* joint movement. The muscle is contracted and movement is opposed by another muscle or by a resistive force. The primary use of this type of exercise is in patients who cannot or should not move their joints, such as those with a joint in a cast or with acute arthritis. Isometric exercise does not require expensive equipment, nor should it be used in patients with diastolic hypertension. Isotonic exercises are strengthening exercises in which the joint is moved through a range of motion against gravity or using weights. Isokinetic exercises are strengthening exercises in which the joint is moved through its range at a constant speed and constant resistance. This type of exercise requires specialized equipment.

408. The answer is D. (*Tollison, p 154.*) Traction is believed to stretch muscles and ligaments, distract vertebral bodies, separate facet joints, and enlarge intervertebral foramina. Contraindications include spinal malignancy, osteomyelitis, bleeding diathesis, osteoporosis, vertebrobasilar insufficiency, severe carotid artery disease, and rheumatoid or inflammatory arthritis. Patients with peptic ulcer, hiatal hernia, or aortic aneurysm should not undergo lumbar traction because of the associated increase in intraabdominal pressure when traction is applied. Cervical traction can be done manually or mechanically with a head harness. The head is maintained at 20 to 25° flexion to open the intervertebral foramina. Weights are added in 2- to 4-kg increments during 20-min sessions over 7 to 10 days until benefit is achieved. Therapy is stopped at a maximum of 22 kg or if no improvement occurs after 7 to 10 sessions. Lumbar traction is exerted via a pelvic harness. A force of 40 kg or more may be needed.

409. The answer is E. (*Raj, pp 934–938.*) Acupuncture has been used for over 2000 years to treat acute and chronic pain. There are 361 classical Chinese acupuncture points, which lie along meridians, extending in a network throughout the body. At the appropriate points, 28- to 30-gauge needles, 1 to 10 cm long, are inserted. Complications of acupuncture include fainting (syncope). Pneumothorax can occur when needles are inserted in the thoracic meridians. Infection can occur if sterile, disposable needles are not used, and needles can break. Electrical current must be used carefully to avoid burns and tissue damage. Massive hemorrhage has not been associated with acupuncture. Some relative contraindications to acupuncture include first-trimester pregnancy (increased risk of spontaneous abortion); rheumatic heart disease (increased risk of endocarditis); anticoagulation (increased risk of localized bleeding); chronic obstructive pulmonary disease (pneumothorax could be catastrophic in these patients); significant psychological overlay (which may make acupuncture therapy unwise); and visceral pain (caution should be used in order to not mask an acute condition).

410. The answer is B. (*Tollison, p 155.*) Massage improves perfusion, facilitates elimination of waste products, reduces soft tissue edema and induration, and can loosen and stretch contracted tissues. Contraindications to massage include infection, inflammatory arthritis, nerve entrapment, phlebitis, and calcification of the soft tissues.

411. The answer is E. (*Tollison, p 156.*) Manipulation is forced, passive movement carrying the articular elements beyond their usual physiologic range of movement. It may be used in the treatment of disorders of the spinal column and peripheral joints. Contraindications include infection, tumor, fracture, vertebrobasilar insufficiency, and gross joint instability. Using manipulation in patients with radicular pain or symptoms of neurologic deficit associated with disk herniation is controversial. Rare cases of vascular insult to the spinal cord or brain as well as the development of radiculopathy have been reported after spinal manipulation.

412. The answer is A. (*Wall, pp 1220–1221.*) The best electrode position for treatment of pain in the lower extremities is the middle to lower thoracic epidural space. For treatment of upper extremity pain, the electrodes should be placed at the high thoracic or low cervical levels. Adjustment should be made during test stimulation to maximize stimulation paresthesias over the painful area without radicular involvement. This patient has left lower extremity pain and would be most likely to benefit from electrodes placed to the left of the physiologic midline of the spinal cord at the level of the middle to lower thoracic vertebrae. In general, stimulation should occur at least one to two and up to four to five segments above the painful dermatomes.

413. The answer is B. (*Wall, p 1222.*) An overall success rate of 61 percent in which patients obtained at least 50 percent relief of their pain symptoms with spinal cord stimulation has been quoted in many studies. Proper patient selection is crucial to successful implantation of a spinal cord stimulator. Patients must be psychologically stable and able to follow instructions. Greatest success has been had with patients suffering from failed back surgery syndrome; postamputation pain; reflex sympathetic dystrophy; brachial, cervical, or lumbar plexopathies; peripheral nerve lesions; and rest pain due to peripheral vascular disease. There is no clear indication for stimulator placement in patients with cancer pain or patients who have had complete transverse lesions of the spinal cord.

414. The answer is D. (*Wall, p 1222.*) Best results occur with spinal cord stimulation when the following protocol is followed:

1. Multipolar electrodes should be used to maximize the area covered and options for different polar combinations.
2. Epidural placement will minimize the risk of cerebrospinal fluid leak.
3. The best placement is at least one to two segments and up to four to five segments above the level of the painful dermatomes.
4. The stimulation paresthesias should cover the painful area as completely as possible and should avoid stimulation of the somatic nerve roots.
5. The patient should have a complete psychological evaluation before trial of spinal cord stimulation. Patients with severe psychological disorders or patients with significant secondary gain from the pain will do poorly with spinal cord stimulation.
6. Pain localized to one area of the body is more easily treated than diffuse pain.

415. The answer is B. (*Bonica, p 1221.*) Eighty-five percent of patients with biliary dyskinesia have relief of pain after endoscopic sphincterotomy. Patients who still have pain after sphincterotomy may benefit from chemical or surgical splanchnicectomy. Blockade of the splanchnic nerves with local anesthetics should be performed (at least twice to document reproducibility of response) prior to undertaking more definitive surgical or neurolytic treatment.

416. The answer is A. (*Bonica, pp 484–487.*) Narcotics administered intramuscularly, intravenously, or by patient-controlled analgesia are the drugs of choice for treatment of acute, severe burn pain and for management of the pain associated with burn therapy. Ketamine used in subanesthetic doses has also provided excellent analgesia for dressing changes and wound debridement. However, tolerance to ketamine develops after repeated use. Silvadine is a topical dressing that prevents dehydration and surface infection and provides some local analgesia. It is not a potent topical anesthetic. Biofeedback and relaxation therapy can significantly reduce self-reported anxiety and burn pain in both adults and children.

417. The answer is B. (*Bonica, p 495.*) The patient has stasis ulcers, most commonly seen in those with chronic venous insufficiency. Treatment consists of elevation of the legs and wearing support stockings. Ulcers can be treated with wet dressings or Unna Boots. If secondary infection is present, the patient should be placed on appropriate antibiotics. Topical steroids may help dermatitis, which can occur from application of other topical ointments, such as neomycin.

418. The answer is D. (*Ramamurthy, p 26.*) PCA pumps are infusion devices interfaced with a microprocessor that controls many infusion parameters. The patient pushes a button connected by a cord to the PCA pump. The pump then records the attempt (button-push) and will release a bolus of medication if an appropriate interval (set dosing interval) has elapsed since the last bolus. The drug is in a syringe in a locked system in the pump. The amount of drug, the dosing interval, the total hourly maximum, and basal infusion rate must be prescribed for each patient. The pump records the total amount of drug used over a period of several hours, and the number of attempts versus the number of actual doses received. This information can be used to maximize analgesia and minimize side effects. Side effects from intravenous narcotics should be managed aggressively.

419. The answer is D. *(Ferrante, p 398.)* A unilateral Horner's syndrome (with resultant miosis) may result during interpleural regional analgesia. Production of Horner's syndrome may be more likely to occur when patients are positioned head down and slightly lateral at the time of injection. Because the patient is still complaining of pain, the next logical step would be to bolus the catheter and then increase the infusion rate.

420. The answer is C. *(Cousins, pp 309–310.)* Motor block is usually assessed by use of the Bromage scale for motor blockade in the lower limbs. Motor blockade in the lower limbs can be assessed with reference to specific myotomes (e.g., L2 hip flexion). A score of 0 is assigned for no block and 1 for complete block (no movement) at each joint on each side.

421. The answer is B. *(Cousins, p 406.)* Stimulation of the radial nerve will yield extension at the elbow, supination of the arm, and extension of the wrist and fingers. Median nerve stimulation produces pronation of the arm; flexion of the wrist; opposition of the middle finger, index finger, and thumb; and flexion of the lateral three fingers. Ulnar nerve stimulation causes flexion of the wrist, adduction of the fingers, and flexion and opposition of the lateral two fingers toward the thumb. Musculocutaneous nerve stimulation causes flexion at the elbow.

422. The answer is E. *(Bonica, pp 1866–1867.)* Side effects and complications associated with dorsal column stimulation are tenderness at the receiver or stimulator site and along the subcutaneous lead, erosion of the skin at the receiver site, dislocation of the electrode, cracks in the lead (which result in leakage of current), bleeding and infection in the epidural space (rare), and infection at the receiver site or along the subcutaneous lead (5 percent). The presence of an epidural mass is a contraindication to placement of a dorsal column stimulator.

423. The answer is D. *(Bonica, p 1934.)* A lumbar sympathetic block will interrupt the sympathetic innervation of the foot, leg and thigh (most commonly ipsilateral; rarely crossover is seen so that sympathetic block on one side results in blockade on the opposite side), urinary bladder, uterus and ovary, testes, epididymis, vas deferens, seminal vesicles, prostate, transverse and descending colon, and rectum. The kidney, adrenal gland, ureter, and ascending colon are innervated by the celiac/splanchnic plexuses.

424. The answer is A. *(Wall, p 1057.)* During a selective posterior rhizotomy, small-diameter primary afferent fibers are preferentially destroyed by a 1- to 2-mm incision in the Lissauer tract, which lies in the ventrolateral aspect of the dorsal rootlet. The large-diameter primary afferent fibers (A-beta) from muscle spindles and proprioceptive afferents enter medial to the small-diameter primary afferent fibers (C and A-delta) and merge in the dorsal column.

425. The answer is E. *(Raj, pp 473–474.)* Intrathecal phenol neurolysis is an appropriate choice for this patient with unilateral cancer pain localized to a few dermatomes. The optimal position for layering of hyperbaric phenol injected intrathecally is for the patient to be tilted backward 45° with the painful side down. This position will increase the likelihood that most of the phenol will bathe the dorsal sensory root rather than the ventral motor root. Phenol is relatively painless on injection and may take 10 to 15 min to fully penetrate the dorsal root. This allows time to make specific adjustments in position over a 10-min period. The patient will note a warm sensation in the areas where phenol has spread. Phenol 4 to 6% in glycerol is very dense. It must be injected through a 20-gauge or larger spinal needle. After injection the patient should be maintained in the optimal position for 45 min before turning.

426. The answer is A. *(Raj, pp 473–474.)* Absolute alcohol is hypobaric to CSF. The patient should be positioned so that the alcohol rises to the top of the CSF in the area of the painful nerve roots. The area of the painful nerve roots should be the highest part of the body so that the alcohol rises as specifically as possible to that area. This may require careful placement of pillows or flexion of the table. Alcohol acts immediately and may be painful on injection. It can be injected through a 25- or 27-gauge spinal needle. After the desired neurolysis is obtained, the patient should remain in position for 45 min.

427. The answer is D. (*Bonica, p 2070.*) Percutaneous C1–C2 cordotomy has been used to successfully treat intractable cancer pain and some malignant pain conditions. A left C1–C2 cordotomy will provide right-sided analgesia below the clavicle to the entire right side except for the right shoulder, which is spared. The procedure is most successful for treatment of lancinating rather than dysesthetic pain. The analgesia can last several months. Complications such as paresis, ataxia, urinary dysfunction, respiratory depression, and dysesthesias occur in 2 to 20 percent of patients. Most complications are temporary, though a small percentage of patients experience permanent side effects after the procedure.

428. The answer is D. (*Tollison, p 387.*) Priapism is an emergency condition in which there is a prolonged, painful penile erection. The patient may require hospitalization and narcotic pain relief as well as sedation. Spinal or caudal anesthesia may cause detumescence. If priapism persists, aspiration of the corpora cavernosa will often be helpful. Surgical shunt of the blood from the corpus cavernosa to the saphenous vein is also successful. Vitamin E and steroid injections can be used as conservative treatment for Peyronie's disease, but not priapism.

429. The answer is A (1,2,3). (*Raj, pp 268–269.*) The sacroiliac joints are true joints consisting of two irregular articulations covered by hyaline cartilage. They are relatively stable, but are weakest anteriorly. Lifting or other movements that involve contraction of the hamstring muscles cause them to be held tight. When lifting and using these muscles for leverage, the sacroiliac joints are most susceptible to injury.

430. The answer is B (1,3). (*Raj, p 868.*) The facet joint and its capsule are richly innervated. Each dorsal ramus sends branches (medial nerve) to the facet joint at its own level and to the level below. Consequently, each posterior ramus innervates two facet joints, and each facet joint has innervation from two levels.

431. The answer is E (all). (*Bonica, pp 2075–2080.*) DREZ lesioning is considered appropriate treatment for brachial plexus lesions (including avulsion), sacral root avulsion, postparaplegic and postquadriplegic pain, phantom limb pain, stump pain, postthoracotomy pain, postherpetic neuralgia, peripheral mononeuropathy, spinal cord tumor, multiple sclerosis, causalgia, and postrhizotomy pain. A well-established diagnosis, failure of medical management, and a patient who is informed of the potential risks are necessary before proceeding with DREZ lesioning. The reported success rate for treatment of brachial plexus avulsion is 83 percent, for postparaplegic or postquadriplegic pain 54 percent, for postamputation pain 39 percent, and for postherpetic neuralgia 59 percent.

432. The answer is B (1,3). (*Cousins, p 1075.*) Cryoanalgesia was introduced to produce destruction of peripheral nerves for the relief of intractable pain that required somatic blockade. Cryolesions are associated with less fibrous tissue reaction than other forms of destruction. The functional loss produced by cryolesioning is associated with a second-degree nerve injury. There is wallerian degeneration with axonal disintegration and breakup of the myelin sheaths, but minimal disruption of the endoneurium and other connective tissue elements. Blockade is based on the Joule-Thompson effect, with nitrous oxide as the refrigerant gas.

433. The answer is A (1,2,3). (*Cousins, p 1056.*) When performing an intrathecal alcohol injection for chest wall pain, the patient should be placed on the table with the affected side upward in the oblique lateral position with the body about 45° to the horizontal. Breaking the table at the proposed injection site assists in maintaining the posterior roots in the uppermost position. To limit the spread of alcohol in the subarachnoid space to the affected segments, the volume of solution injected should be small and the rate of injection slow.

434. The answer is A (1,2,3). (*Cousins, p 948.*) Clinical studies have shown that epidural steroids do depress plasma cortisol levels for about 2 weeks, but clinical manifestations of systemic side effects have been uncommon. These include congestive heart failure owing to fluid retention, minor changes in serum glucose level in susceptible patients, cramps, rash, malaise, fever, and digestive problems.

435. The answer is C (2,4). *(Cousins, p 937.)* The medial branches of the lumbar dorsal rami emerge from respective intertransverse spaces, and each nerve crosses the upper border of the lower transverse process. Articular branches are given off to the zygapophysial facet joints above and below the nerve, and eventually each medial branch enters the mutifidus muscle. Each lumbar zygapophysial facet joint is supplied by at least two nerves: the medial branch above its location and the one below. Therefore, a given joint can be substantially, if not completely, anesthetized by blocking these two nerves.

436. The answer is E (all). *(Cousins, p 923.)* Intercostal nerve block is one of the most useful procedures for relief of a severe, acute, posttraumatic, postoperative, or postinfectious pain in the thoracic or abdominal wall. It is highly effective in relieving severe pain resulting from fracture of one or more ribs or the sternum, dislocation of the costochondral junction, slipped rib cartilage, contusion chest pain, pleurisy, and acute herpes zoster. It is a useful therapeutic procedure in entrapment of the intercostal nerves in the rectus sheath, which is said to be a frequent cause of abdominal and chest pain.

437. The answer is E (all). *(Cousins, p 900.)* Neurogenic pain syndromes in which local anesthetic nerve blocks may be useful include neuralgias of the cranial and spinal nerves; radiculopathies of cervical and lumbar nerve roots; cervical, brachial, and lumbosacral plexalgias; peripheral neuralgias and neuropathies (diabetic, nutritional); and compression and entrapment syndromes.

438. The answer is A (1,2,3). *(Cousins, p 732.)* The anatomic position of the celiac plexus renders it susceptible to many hazards from nerve block. Possible sequelae from accidental subarachnoid injection include lower extremity weakness, paralysis, and loss of function of the anal and bladder sphincters. Hypotension commonly follows celiac plexus block. It results from interruption of vasoconstrictor fibers in the viscera and omentum. Bowel motility is commonly increased during the first few days after the block, but gradually returns to normal.

439. The answer is B (1,3). *(Cousins, p 699.)* Situations in which high venous pressure is likely to occur during intravenous Bier block include performing a rapid injection, injecting into a proximal vein, injecting a large volume of solution, and inadequate exsanguination of the extremity. As venous pressure increases, leakage of injectate proximal to the pneumatic cuffs is more likely to occur.

440. The answer is C (2,4). *(Cousins, p 657.)* The ilioinguinal nerve, which has its origins from T12 and, more particularly, L1, is readily blocked as it passes close to the prominent anterior superior iliac spine. It lies deep to the fascia of the external oblique muscle and emerges with the spermatic cord through the external inguinal ring to continue to the penoscrotal area in the male or the labial area in the female.

441. The answer is B (1,3). *(Cousins, p 685.)* The common peroneal nerve leaves the tibial nerve at the apex of the popliteal fossa and runs laterally just medial to the biceps femoris muscle and deep to the popliteal fascia. It should not be blocked as it passes around the neck of the fibula, since neuralgia is more likely to occur.

442. The answer is E (all). *(Cousins, 551.)* A deep cervical plexus block is, in effect, a paravertebral nerve block of C2–4 spinal nerves as they emerge from the foramina in the cervical vertebrae. The sites of needle insertion are located by reference to a line that joins the tip of the mastoid process with the C6 transverse process (Chassaignac's tubercle), which is palpated at the level of the cricoid cartilage. The C4 needle insertion site is approximated by drawing a horizontal line through the lower border of the ramus of the mandible to intersect this line.

443. The answer is A (1,2,3). *(Cousins pp 572–573.)* An inferior alveolar nerve block is used to provide hard tissue anesthesia from the mandible to the midline and labial soft tissue anesthesia from the bicuspid teeth to the midline. For complete anesthesia of the mandible, this block must be supplemented with long buccal and lingual nerve blocks. The masseter nerve is a motor branch of the anterior division of the mandibular nerve.

444. The answer is E (all). *(Cousins, p 551.)* The cervical plexus is distributed to the skin of the anterolateral neck by way of the anterior primary rami of C2–4. These emerge as four distinct nerves, the lesser occipital, greater auricular, anterior cervical, and supraclavicular nerves. All four branches can be blocked by infiltration at the midpoint of the posterior sternocleidomastoid muscle.

445. The answer is A (1,2,3). *(Cousins, p 551.)* The greater occipital nerve is best blocked as it crosses the superior nuchal line, about one-third of the way between the external occipital protuberance and the mastoid process. It is located at this site by palpating the occipital artery that lies adjacent to it.

446. The answer is A (1,2,3). *(Cousins, p 551.)* An accessory nerve block can be used for trapezius muscle block as an adjunct to interscalene nerve blocks of the brachial plexus for surgery on the shoulder. By blocking the accessory nerve in the posterior triangle of the neck, the trapezius muscle is paralyzed and surgery is often facilitated. The accessory nerve lies superficial to the prevertebral fascia and so lies deep only to skin, platysma muscle, and deep cervical fascia. Therefore, if a needle is introduced at the junction of the middle and superior thirds of the sternocleidomastoid muscle at its lateral border, and local anesthetic is injected, an accessory nerve block can be accomplished.

447. The answer is E (all). *(Cousins, p 547.)* Glossopharyngeal nerve block is used most frequently for inoperable carcinomas that invade the distribution of the nerve in either the posterior third of the tongue or the pharyngeal areas. Possible sequelae include unilateral blockade of the accessory nerve with resulting weakness of the sternocleidomastoid and trapezius muscles, numbness of the laryngeal inlet and trachea, and paralysis of the ipsilateral vocal cords with resulting hoarseness.

448. The answer is A (1,2,3). *(Cousins, p 547.)* In the performance of a glossopharyngeal nerve block, a needle is inserted at the midpoint of a line joining the angle of the mandible to the tip of the mastoid process of the occipital bone. The needle is advanced medially. Ideally, the styloid process is located as the bony landmark, which allows adjustment of the needle posterior to the process but at the same depth as the process.

449. The answer is B (1,3). *(Cousins, p 546.)* The glossopharyngeal nerve (CN IX) emerges via the jugular foramen, in close proximity to the vagus (CN X) and accessory (CN XI) nerves, along with the internal jugular vein. It is blocked just below this point, and therefore both temporary and permanent blocks usually involve the other two cranial nerves, all three of which lie in the groove between the internal jugular vein and the internal carotid artery.

450. The answer is E (all). *(Cousins, p 545.)* Using a lateral approach, the maxillary nerve can be blocked as it crosses the pterygopalatine fossa. A needle is inserted below the midpoint of the zygomatic arch overlying the coronoid notch of the mandible. As the needle passes through the subcutaneous tissue (which contains the parotid gland), it is directed medially until it reaches the medial wall of the infratemporal fossa, where it will strike the lateral surface of the lateral pterygoid plate. From this point, the needle is "walked" anteriorly until it reaches the pterygopalatine fossa. Because of the highly vascular nature of the contents of the fossa (maxillary artery), a hematoma frequently occurs after this block.

451. The answer is B (1,3). *(Cousins, p 543.)* The nasociliary nerve divides into its terminal branches, anterior ethmoidal and infratrochlear nerves, on the medial wall of the orbit 2.5 cm from the orbital margin. Both branches are blocked by inserting a 5-cm, 25-gauge needle 1 cm above the inner canthus. The needle is directed backward and slightly medially to pass just lateral to the inner wall of the orbit and medial to the eyeball and medial rectus muscle. The depth of insertion is 2.5 cm, and at this point 1 mL of 2% lidocaine or an equivalent local anesthetic is injected as the needle is slowly withdrawn.

452. The answer is A (1,2,3). *(Cousins, p 542.)* The supraorbital nerve, like the infraorbital and mental nerves, lies in the same vertical plane as the pupil when the patient is looking straight ahead. The supratrochlear nerve is a terminal branch of the ophthalmic division of the trigeminal nerve that supplies the forehead. It emerges from the superomedial angle of the orbit.

453. The answer is E (all). (*Cousins, p 398.*) In the performance of an interscalene block, the patient's head is temporarily lifted in order to palpate the posterior border of the sternocleidomastoid muscle. The interscalene groove is palpated by rolling the fingers from the border of the sternocleidomastoid, over the belly of the scalenus anterior, and into the interscalene groove. A line is then extended directly laterally from the cricoid cartilage to intersect the interscalene groove. The point of entry is at the process of C6. The external jugular vein may overlie this point.

454. The answer is C (2,4). (*Cousins, p 431.*) Distally, the anterior branch of the obturator nerve supplies an articular branch to the hip joint, the anterior adductor muscle, and cutaneous branches to the lower inner thigh. The presence of successful obturator nerve block is determined by demonstrating paresis of the adductor muscle since the cutaneous distribution is small and inconstant.

455. The answer is E (all). (*Cousins, pp 429–430.*) Several techniques have been described for performing a lateral femoral cutaneous nerve block. After palpating the anterior superior iliac spine, a point 2 to 3 cm inferior and 2 to 3 cm medial is marked. The needle is advanced posteriorly through the fascia lata, where the injection is performed. Alternatively, the needle can be directed slightly lateral and cephalad to strike the iliac bone just medial and below the anterior superior iliac spine, where the nerve emerges. The lateral femoral cutaneous nerve can also be blocked by inserting a short, beveled needle just medial to the anterior superior iliac spine and advancing it until a "pop" is felt as the needle passes through the external oblique aponeurosis. A second "pop" is felt after penetration of the internal oblique muscle and underlying fascia iliaca.

456. The answer is B (1,3). (*Cousins, pp 425–427.*) The classic approach to the sciatic nerve block is with the patient lying on the side opposite the one to be blocked and rolled forward onto the flexed knee with the heel in opposition to the knee of the outstretched dependent leg. Landmarks used for performing a classic sciatic block include the greater trochanter of the femur, the posterior superior iliac spine, the piriformis muscle, and the sacrosciatic foramen. Anterior, lithotomy, and lateral approaches to performing a sciatic nerve block have also been described.

457. The answer is A (1,2,3). (*Cousins, p 423.*) Since the sacral nerves represent the parasympathetic portion of the autonomic nervous system, sympathetic blockade with its potential for hypotension is not seen with transsacral block unless excessive volumes of solution spread proximally to the lumbar sympathetic fibers. However, loss of parasympathetic function to bowel, bladder, and sphincters may occur. Injection of local anesthetic through misdirected needles into the subarachnoid or vascular compartments is a remote risk.

458. The answer is B (1,3). (*Cousins, p 423.*) For transsacral block, the patient is placed prone over a pillow placed under the hips. The posterior superior iliac spine and sacral cornu are both palpated and marked. Points are marked 1 cm medial to and below the posterior superior iliac spine and immediately lateral to and above the sacral cornu. The distance between these two points is dissected and a third point is marked. The three points identify the second, third, and fourth sacral foramina.

459. The answer is B (1,3). (*Cousins, p 420.*) The lumbar plexus lies between the quadratus lumborum muscle posteriorly and the psoas major muscle anteriorly; it is invested by the fasciae of these two muscles. Although the other nerves to the leg take divergent courses through the plexus, the femoral nerve descends from under the psoas muscle and remains in the groove of the psoas and iliacus muscles.

460. The answer is A (1,2,3). (*Cousins, p 413.*) The thumb is supplied by superficial branches of the radial nerve and by digital branches of the median nerve. Thus, complete sensory block of the thumb is produced by median and radial nerve blocks at the wrist. The thumb can also be blocked by circumferential infiltration at the base of the thumb ("ring" block) using a solution that does not contain epinephrine.

MEDICAL AND SURGICAL TECHNIQUES OF PAIN MANAGEMENT *ANSWERS*

461. The answer is A (1,2,3). (*Cousins, p 411.*) There are three described techniques to successfully block the musculocutaneous nerve. First, it may be blocked at the main nerve trunk in the substance of the coracobrachialis muscle. Second, it may be blocked 5 cm proximal to the elbow crease, where the terminal sensory lateral cutaneous nerve of the forearm emerges from between the brachialis and biceps muscles. Third, the block can be performed just lateral to the tendon of the biceps muscle at the level of the intercondylar line. The median nerve is typically blocked just medial to the brachial artery along the intercondylar line.

462. The answer is C (2,4). (*Cousins, p 411.*) Radial nerve block at the wrist is a field block of the superficial terminal branches as they pass in a variable manner over the radial side of the carpus. The "anatomic snuffbox," which is made prominent by extension of the thumb, serves as the landmark for performing this block. It is found between the extensor pollicis longus and brevis tendons.

463. The answer is A (1,2,3). (*Cousins, pp 407–410.*) The radial nerve is blocked at the level of the elbow as it passes over the anterior aspect of the lateral epicondyle of the humerus. Prior to needle insertion, the intercondylar line is marked and the biceps tendon is palpated. From a point along the intercondylar line, 2 cm lateral to the biceps tendon, a needle is advanced posteriorly to contact the surface of the lateral epicondyle approximating the radial nerve. The brachial artery is an important landmark when performing a median nerve block at the elbow.

464. The answer is B (1,3). (*Cousins, pp 408–409.*) At the wrist, the ulnar nerve is blocked where it lies under the flexor carpi ulnaris tendon just proximal to the pisiform bone, before it bifurcates into deep (motor) and superficial (sensory) terminal branches. At this point, the nerve lies lateral and deep to the ulnar artery.

465. The answer is E (all). (*Cousins, p 400.*) The phrenic nerve is frequently blocked because of C4 root involvement or because of anterior spread of local anesthetic under the prevertebral fascia in front of the scalenus anterior muscle. However, this is seldom significant in unilateral blocks. Vagus, recurrent laryngeal, and cervical sympathetic nerves are sometimes involved, but are of no clinical significance except that it may be important to reassure the patient if side effects develop.

466. The answer is E (all). (*Cousins, p 398.*) Phrenic nerve block occurs in 40 to 60 percent of cases and usually causes no symptoms. Horner's syndrome occurs in approximately 70 to 90 percent of brachial plexus blocks when large volumes of solution are used. The symptoms resolve as the block dissipates, and no treatment is necessary. Nerve damage or neuritis is an uncommon but possible complication of all peripheral blocks, including the supraclavicular technique for blocking the brachial plexus. The most common reason for the occurrence of a toxic reaction to local anesthetic drugs is an unintentional intravascular injection or use of an excessive amount of solution.

467. The answer is B (1,3). (*Cousins, p 396.*) The most specific complication of the supraclavicular approach for blocking the brachial plexus is a pneumothorax. The frequency of occurrence is between 0.5 and 6 percent. Tall, thin patients (who characteristically have high apical pleurae) usually account for a greater number of these complications. The risk of pneumothorax can be minimized by using fine, short needles. The majority of cases take up to 24 h to become clinically significant. They are usually small to moderate in size and may or may not cause symptoms that require further medical or surgical interventions (such as a chest tube).

468. The answer is B (1,3). (*Cousins, p 374.*) Many factors have been implicated in influencing the spread of a standard dose of local anesthetic solution injected into the caudal canal. Such factors as age, weight, height, dose, and speed of injection will be known or controllable. The only two factors that have been shown to affect caudal spread in adults are dose and speed of injection.

469. The answer is C (2,4). (*Cousins, p 374.*) Confirmation of bony landmarks is the key to success for a caudal block. The posterior superior iliac spines form an equilateral triangle with the sacral hiatus. This should be used as a confirmatory landmark for correct needle placement. In thin, young patients, the protrusions of the sacral cornua can be seen without palpation, and the shallow depression over the sacral hiatus can be seen between them.

470. **The answer is E (all).** (*Cousins, p 393.*) There are several advantages to the use of the supraclavicular block. The brachial plexus is blocked where it is most compactly arranged—at the level of the three trunks. A low volume of solution is required, and quick onset is achieved. Also, the technique can be performed with the arm in virtually any position, and all the brachial plexus is reliably blocked.

471. **The answer is A (1,2,3).** (*Cousins, p 395.*) Landmarks used for performing a supraclavicular brachial plexus block include the clavicular head of the sternocleidomastoid muscle, which helps in identifying the interscalene groove. Because the brachial plexus makes its exit at the lateral border of the anterior scalene muscle, the skin is marked at this point, immediately above the clavicle. The subclavian artery can often be palpated in the supraclavicular fossa because it also emerges from the lower end of the interscalene groove. This serves as a check on the other landmarks. An additional guide to locating the midpoint of the clavicle is finding the point where the straight portion of the external jugular vein, if continued, would cross the clavicle.

472. **The answer is D (4).** (*Cousins, p 1077.*) Hypophysectomy relieves pain in a similar percentage (60 to 90 percent) of cancer patients, regardless of whether it is carried out surgically by transcranial or open microsurgical technique, by transnasal cryoprobe, or by transnasal alcohol injection. The characteristics of the pain relief are also similar, regardless of how the hypophysectomy is performed. In those who respond, onset of relief is rapid, occurring within minutes to hours of the procedure, and is usually complete.

473. **The answer is E (all).** (*Cousins, p 123.*) As the dose and blood levels of lidocaine are increased, a prolongation of conduction time through various parts of the heart occurs, which is seen on the ECG as an increase in the PR interval and QRS duration. Extremely high concentrations of local anesthetic may result in sinus bradycardia and sinus arrest. A similar depression at the AV node also occurs, resulting in prolonged PR intervals and partial and complete AV dissociation.

474. **The answer is B (1,3).** (*Bonica, p 1653.*) Opioid-induced itching is believed to be a centrally mediated phenomenon that is more severe with intraspinal opioids than oral opioids. The itching is usually most prominent in the face and trunk. Low-dose naloxone (an opioid antagonist) can decrease the itching without significantly decreasing opioid-induced analgesia. Nalbuphine is a mu-receptor agonist and kappa-receptor antagonist that has also been used to relieve opioid-induced pruritus. Diphenhydramine (Benadryl) can also decrease the severity of the itching. The mechanism of action for this effect is unknown. Naltrexone is a long-acting mu-receptor antagonist used in opioid addiction control programs. Hydroxyzine (Vistaril) increases the analgesic effect of morphine by at least 50 percent and is a potent antiemetic. It has no effect on opioid-induced pruritus.

475. **The answer is E (all).** (*Ferrante, p 396.*) Interpleural analgesia is an effective method of postoperative pain management after unilateral surgical incisions in the chest or abdomen. Cholecystectomy, mastectomy, and nephrectomy are the surgical procedures most effectively treated with interpleural analgesia. Also, the pain from pancreatic cancer can be relieved using an interpleural technique by diffusion of the local anesthetic through the pleura to reach the celiac plexus.

476. **The answer is A (1,2,3).** (*Raj, pp 787–788.*) Interrruption of sympathetic nerves to the head, supplied by the stellate ganglion, can be easily documented by the presence of Horner's syndrome: miosis (pinpoint pupil), ptosis (drooping of the upper eyelid), and enophthalmos (sinking of the eyeball). Associated findings include conjunctival injection, nasal congestion, and facial anhidrosis. These signs can be present without complete interruption of the sympathetic nerves to the upper extremity.

477. **The answer is C (2,4).** (*Cousins, pp 405–406.*) When using a nerve stimulator to perform a peripheral nerve block, it is vital that a motor response be obtained at only minimal current output, approximately 0.1 mA. Otherwise, the tip of the needle may be still some distance from the nerve. Although uninsulated needles can at times be successfully used, accuracy increases with coated needles. The cathode (−) of the stimulator must be attached to the needle; otherwise, four times as much current is needed to stimulate the nerve.

478. The answer is A (1,2,3). (*Cousins, p 273.*) In the lumbar region, the major cause of a negative pressure lies in "coning" of the dura by the advancing needle point. By this means, negative pressure increases as the needle advances across the epidural space toward the dura. Blunt needles with side openings produce greater negative pressure as does slow introduction of the needle. Greater negative pressure can also be obtained if the dura is not distended (e.g., by gravity in the sitting position or by high abdominal or thoracic pressure).

479. The answer is B (1,3). (*Raj, pp 474–475.*) Indications for epidural neurolysis include pain in the shoulder or upper extremities, the thoracic wall and pleura, and the upper abdominal wall. The advantage of epidural neurolysis over intrathecal neurolysis is that the positioning is not so critical and that neurolysis can be carried out over a period of 2 to 3 days by intermittent injection of phenol or alcohol through the epidural catheter. Baricity, which is the weight of the agent in relation to the weight of CSF, is paramount in neurolytic intrathecal injection. It plays little or no role, however, in a neurolytic block in the epidural space.

480. The answer is E (all). (*Raj, p 763.*) Symptoms resulting from a subdural injection of local anesthetic result from the small volume space as well as the location of trabeculae and extension of the subdural space into the cranium. There is usually a delay of up to 10 to 20 min before onset of symptoms after a subdural injection. The symptoms of unexpected, widespread, sensory and motor blockade occur after a negative aspiration test and with what would be considered normal doses for epidural injection. The pattern of blockade can be patchy and unilateral in nature. Because of extension into the cranium, spread of local anesthetics can manifest effects on cranial nerves. The duration of symptoms caused by subdural injection is more similar to that of an epidural than an intrathecal injection.

481. The answer is A (1,2,3). (*Cousins, pp 585–586.*) Akinesia of the extraocular muscles during a retrobulbar injection is provided by blockade of cranial nerves III, IV, and VI. Cranial nerve VII (facial nerve) can be blocked by any one of several extraocular techniques. The most common technique, the classic Van Lint approach, blocks the facial nerve at the lateral orbital rim.

482. The answer is B (1,3). (*Raj, p 74.*) Therapeutic interventions that may possibly provide some relief in neuropathic pain syndromes include neural blockade and administration of narcotics, anxiolytics, antidepressants, and anticonvulsants. Anti-inflammatory agents as well as further neurologic damage (surgical) usually are not effective.

483. The answer is D (4). (*Raj, p 75.*) Therapeutic modalities that may be useful in treating intractable chronic pain include antidepressants, cognitive coping strategies, and behavior modification. Anti-inflammatory agents are unlikely to be effective and narcotics as well as sedative-hypnotics are relatively contraindicated. Neural blockade, when performed in patients with intractable chronic pain, is unpredictable and usually ineffective.

484. The answer is A (1,2,3). (*Raj, p 76.*) Any sympathetic block interrupts both afferent and efferent activity; indeed, the measure of a successful sympathetic blockade is a rise in temperature (indicating blockade of efferent vasoconstrictor fibers). It is theoretically possible that pain relief is secondary to the increased blood flow and not indicative of sympathetically maintained pain. Conversely, a somatic nerve block also interrupts the sympathetic fibers traveling in that nerve.

485. The answer is E (all). (*Raj, p 581.*) Initial treatment of coccygodynia involves using cushions or rubber doughnuts to redistribute the weight and relieve the pressure on the coccyx while the patient is sitting. Caudal epidural steroid injections as well as neurolytic techniques directed toward the fourth and fifth sacral nerves have also been reported to provide pain relief from coccygodynia. Surgical alternatives consist of coccygectomy and surgical rhizotomy of the lower sacral roots.

486. The answer is A (1,2,3). (*Wall, p 893.*) TENS has provided long-lasting relief in a small number of patients with central poststroke pain syndrome. It is most successful in patients who have not lost the sense of touch and vibration. Antidepressants and antiepileptic drugs have also been helpful. Peripheral neurolysis is not helpful. Treatment should be tailored to address the particular constellation of pain symptoms in each patient. In general, this is a very difficult condition to treat.

487. The answer is E (all). (*Tollison, p 137.*) Relative contraindications include patients with demand-type cardiac pacemakers; electrode placement over the eye, carotid sinus, heart, or pregnant uterus; placement on the head in epileptics or stroke patients; placement on mucous membranes; patients with allergy to electrode adhesive; and patients with dementia or other psychiatric disorders.

488. The answer is E (all). (*Tollison, pp 140–141.*) Deep brain stimulation is a reversible, nonablative procedure that can be used to treat central deafferentation pain states. It is especially useful in patients in whom spinal cord stimulation or peripheral nerve stimulation has failed. Placement is done stereotactically under local anesthesia. Usually two electrodes are placed in the bilateral periaqueductal gray/periventricular gray (PAG/PVG) in patients with midline or bilateral pain. In patients with unilateral deafferentation pain, one electrode is placed in the contralateral PAG/PVG and another in the contralateral sensory thalamus (ventroposterolateral or ventroposteromedial nuclei). If trial stimulation is successful, the electrodes can be connected to subcutaneously implanted electronics under general anesthesia. Indications include deafferentation pain syndromes treated by thalamic electrode placement (thalamic syndrome, anesthesia dolorosa, postherpetic neuralgia, phantom limb, postcordotomy dysesthesia, pain of spinal cord injury, brachial or lumbosacral plexus avulsions, chronic lumbosacral radiculopathy). Pain responsive to narcotics can be treated by PAG electrode placement (chronic low back pain or leg pain not due to radiculopathy or deafferentation, cancer pain not due to nerve infiltration, nonmalignant abdominal or perineal pain, atypical facial pain). Complications include intracranial hemorrhage (2 to 4 percent), infection (3 to 6 percent), eye movement abnormalities (2 to 4 percent), and hardware failures (2 to 12 percent). The fatality rate is less than 2 percent.

489. The answer is E (all). (*Barolat, Stereotact Funct Neurosurg 56:77–103, 1991. Broseta, J Neurosurg 64:71–80, 1986. North, Neurosurgery 32:384–395, 1993.*) SCS can be used to effectively treat peripheral deafferentation pain such as postamputation neuralgia (stump pain), intractable neuralgia, and unilateral cervical or lumbosacral radiculitis. It can also be used to treat reflex sympathetic dystrophy (most successful in patients with involvement of a single extremity), phantom limb pain, and postherpetic neuralgia. One of the most common indications for insertion of the SCS in Europe is vasculopathic (ischemic) pain. Bilateral pain syndromes (e.g., bilateral RSD or failed back surgery syndrome) can be treated with SCS, but the technical complexity is increased and a significant amount of experience with implantation is required to assure successful patient selection and good outcome. The overall, long-term success rate (> 50 percent pain relief for > 7 years) is approximately 50 percent.

490. The answer is E (all). (*Tollison, p 158.*) Low-power cold laser therapy does not produce irreversible tissue damage. It may relieve pain by decreasing arteriolar spasm, exciting mitochondrial membranes, enhancing activity of superoxide dismutase, and increasing levels of serum serotonin. So far, no known contraindications or side effects have been noted. Care should be taken in use on pregnant patients or patients with malignancy. Protective eye wear is necessary. Staring directly into the beam may cause retinal damage.

491. The answer is C (2,4). (*Bonica, p 1777.*) Iontophoresis, or ion transfer, involves applying an electrical current of low intensity to a tissue as an electromotive force to induce chemical changes. These changes result in increased blood flow, whereby substances can then be introduced in order to accentuate the healing process (e.g., zinc oxide into decubitus ulcers). Positive ions and alkaloids are driven into the skin at the anode; negative ions and acidoids are driven into the skin at the cathode.

492. The answer is B (1,3). (*Raj, pp 670–671.*) Superficial heating modalities include hot packs (hydrocollator therapy), paraffin bath, fluidotherapy, hydrotherapy, and radiant heat. These heating modalities are applied only to the skin and subcutaneous tissue and usually do not produce heat beyond the depth of 1 cm. Ultrasound and short-wave diathermy are considered *deep* heating modalities and can heat structures to a depth of 3 to 5 cm.

493. The answer is B (1,3). (*Raj, p 287.*) Facet joint pain may be relieved by denervating the joint or blocking the nerve that supplies the joint. The nerve that innervates the joint comes from the corresponding nerve root and another branch from one level above. Blockade is commonly performed by placing a needle or cryoprobe at the junction of the superior facet and the transverse process at each level.

494. The answer is E (all). (*Ready, p 7.*) Four principles should be applied to all plans for therapy of acute pain:

1. The source and degree of painful stimuli should be determined
2. The relationship between nociception and other aspects of suffering—such as anxiety, cultural variation, or response to pain and the meaning of pain (malignant versus benign disease)—should be understood and treated as necessary.
3. Drug levels should be adequate to provide sufficient analgesia to perform the activities needed for healing.
4. Therapy should be frequently evaluated and adjusted to provide optimal analgesia for the individual patient.

495. The answer is A (1,2,3). (*Cousins, p 408.*) When performing a median nerve block at the elbow, the arm is positioned abducted on a board with the elbow extended and the forearm supinated. The intercondylar line between medial and lateral epicondyles of the humerus is drawn across the cubital fossa and the brachial artery is palpated and marked at this level. The needle is inserted just medial to the artery perpendicular to the skin, and the block is performed after a paresthesia is elicited.

496. The answer is A (1,2,3). (*Raj, p 709.*) Cryolesioning involves using a probe tip cooled to –60°C (–76°F) to produce lesions of various nerves involved in transmitting painful impulses. After a nerve is frozen, axonal disintegration, wallerian degeneration, and disruption of the myelin sheath occur. However, the integrity of the Schwann cell basal lamina remains intact, providing a conduit for regeneration of nerve fiber. Freezing causes severe injury to all nerve fibers, which persists for 1 to 2 months before regeneration begins.

497. The answer is A (1,2,3). (*Cousins, p 517.*) The easiest approach to the well-guarded celiac plexus is posterolateral, using the 12th ribs and the inferior aspects of the T12 and L1 spinous processes as external landmarks. The figure formed by connecting the spinous processes of T12 and L1 with points 7 to 8 cm lateral at the lower edges of both 12th ribs is a flattened isosceles triangle. Local anesthetic should be injected at the point 7 to 8 cm lateral to the most distal aspect of the L1 spinous process to anesthetize skin and subcutaneous tissues. Under fluoroscopic guidance, a 12- to 15-cm, 20- to 22-gauge needle should then be inserted at a 40 to 45° angle until the celiac plexus is reached.

498. The answer is A (1,2,3). (*Tollison, pp 174–175.*) Hypnosis can be a useful adjunctive pain treatment for patients with acute and chronic pain. It has been used to decrease the pain of both adult and pediatric burn patients undergoing daily tanking, debridement, and dressing changes. It can also be used to treat headaches, back pain, cancer pain, phantom limb pain, facial pain, neck and shoulder pain, myofibrositis, herpes, lupus, GI pain, bruxism, tick douloureux, vaginismus, arthritis, and peripheral nerve pain.

The patient's ability to experience decreased pain through hypnosis in acute and chronic pain states is directly related to the patient's level of hypnotic susceptibility. Hypnosis reduces both the sensation of pain and the suffering components of pain and is not due to placebo effect. For patients with low susceptibility to hypnosis, the reduction of pain is not greater than with placebo. However, for patients with high susceptibility to hypnosis, pain reduction under hypnosis is much greater than that experienced with placebo.

499. The answer is B (1,3). (*Capan, p 694.*) In normovolemic patients, blockade to T6 does not cause significant hemodynamic changes. Lower extremity vessels dilate and upper extremity vessels constrict, thereby maintaining total systemic vascular resistance. Blockade to T3–T4 will decrease total systemic vascular resistance by 15 to 20 percent, increase cardiac output by 15 to 20 percent, and have little effect on mean arterial pressure. Blockade limited to T3–T12 will decrease mean arterial pressure by 10 to 15 percent because of reduced total systemic vascular resistance. The 10 percent reduction in heart rate that occurs is counteracted by a 10 percent increase in stroke volume. Therefore, there is no change in cardiac output. In hypovolemic patients with blockade to T4–T5, severe reductions in heart rate, mean arterial pressure, and cardiac output can occur. The hypotension may be severe enough to cause cardiac arrest.

500. The answer is A (1,2,3). (*Bonica, p 1934.*) The cervicothoracic (stellate) sympathetic ganglion can be blocked by 15 to 20 mL of local anesthetic, which spreads in the proper fascial plane to involve the sympathetic chain from the lower portion of the superior cervical ganglion to the T5 ganglion. This blocks the sympathetic fibers to the head and neck, upper extremities, the heart, and most of the fibers to the lungs and esophagus. A celiac-splanchnic block would be required to block the sympathetic innervation of the stomach.

501. The answer is C (2,4). (*Bonica, p 1934.*) Injection of 15 to 25 mL of local anesthetic bilaterally, anterior to the vertebral body of L1, will block all the sympathetic and vagal efferent and afferent fibers from the viscera in the upper abdomen. This includes the stomach, small intestine, liver, gallbladder, pancreas, spleen, adrenal glands, ureters, kidney, ascending colon, and transverse colon. The rectum and descending colon sympathetics are blocked when a lumbar sympathetic block is performed.

502. The answer is D (4). (*Tollison, pp 480–481.*) Osteoarthritis is a chronic degenerative disease associated with cartilage breakdown, sclerosis of subchondral bone, and osteophyte formation. There is no cure for the disease; therefore, treatment of symptoms is the cornerstone of management. Drug therapy consists of salicylates or NSAIDS and acetaminophen with codeine or propoxyphene as needed. These drugs do not have any effect on the underlying disease process, but are useful for pain relief. Intraarticular corticosteroids can be used to treat articular pain unresponsive to NSAIDS. Injections should not be administered more frequently than once every 4 months. Repeat injections should not be performed unless the patient gets more than 4 weeks of relief. Physical therapy is helpful, as is weight reduction and the use of assistive devices such as canes, walkers, and crutches to help relieve pain due to weight-bearing on arthritic joints. However, comprehensive physical therapy programs can be expensive, and there is poor patient compliance with outpatient exercise programs.

503. The answer is B (1,3). (*Tollison, 167–172.*) Contraindications to spinal manipulation include cervical osteophytes, which may obstruct the vertebral arteries during manipulation, and cervical degenerative joint disease with diminished disk height, which allows the vertebral arteries to become more tortuous and places them at risk for obstruction or injury during manipulation. Sixty-two percent of patients with fixed posterior lumbar facet syndrome found spinal manipulation to be beneficial. Spondylolisthesis is not a contraindication to spinal manipulation and can be beneficial in some cases. Manipulation is most successful if directed to the sacroiliac joints or posterior joints above the level of the slippage in cases of L4 or L5 spondylolisthesis.

504. The answer is A (1,2,3). (*Bonica, p 1290.*) The superior, middle, and inferior hypogastric plexi contain the sympathetic and parasympathetic nerves, which innervate the pelvic viscera. The superior hypogastric plexus is formed by union of the branches of the aortic plexus and the L3 and L4 splanchnic nerves. The inferior mesenteric plexus supplies the pelvic portion of the large bowel.

505. The answer is E (all). (*Tollison, p 387.*) In phimosis the foreskin cannot be retracted without significant pain and tenderness. In paraphimosis the retracted foreskin forms a constricting band at the base of the glans. Chronic irritation of the glans penis caused by the foreskin is called *balanitis*. Condyloma acuminata (genital warts) can form under the foreskin and the infection can spread. Carcinoma of the penis is virtually nonexistent in males who were circumcised at birth, but does occur in uncircumcised males. Recommended treatment for the above conditions is circumcision.

Pain Management in the Pediatric, Critical Care, and Obstetric Populations

DIRECTIONS: Each question below contains suggested responses. Select the **one best** response.

506. The analogue chromatic continuous scale (ACCS) allows a child to rate his or her pain according to

    (A) numbers
    (B) faces
    (C) color
    (D) words
    (E) pictures

507. A 32-year-old woman who had epidural analgesia (bupivacaine and morphine) for vaginal delivery of a 9-lb, 6-oz baby boy complains of numbness and footdrop 24 h after delivery. The most likely cause is

    (A) transient neurologic deficit due to compression of the nerves by the baby during delivery
    (B) permanent neuropathy from pelvic neural compression
    (C) herniated intervertebral disk
    (D) ischemia of the conus medullaris
    (E) myelopathy due to epidural analgesia

508. Pain assessment and measurement in children between the ages of 2 and 7 years is best evaluated by

    (A) visual analogue scale rating
    (B) body movements and facial expressions
    (C) self-report
    (D) Oucher scale (faces scale)

509. Which of the following statements is true regarding the effect of spinally administered narcotic agents on pain and the stress response?

    (A) They completely block the stress response to surgery
    (B) Plasma glucose and cortisol levels are lower than in patients receiving general anesthesia and parenteral narcotics
    (C) Plasma glucose and cortisol levels are lower than in patients receiving epidural local anesthetics
    (D) They suppress the pain pathways involving gamma-aminobutyric acid and the sympathetic afferents
    (E) They block A-beta and A-delta neural fibers preferentially

510. Which of the following is NOT recommended to provide sedation and reduce anxiety in critically ill patients in an intensive care setting?

    (A) Morphine
    (B) Hydromorphone
    (C) Midazolam
    (D) Etomidate
    (E) Lorazepam

DIRECTIONS: Each question below contains four suggested responses of which **one or more** is correct. Select

A	if	**1, 2, and 3**	are correct
B	if	**1 and 3**	are correct
C	if	**2 and 4**	are correct
D	if	**4**	is correct
E	if	**1, 2, 3, and 4**	are correct

511. Advantages of acetaminophen over aspirin when used as an analgesic in children include

    (1) lack of gastric irritation
    (2) no association with Reye syndrome
    (3) lack of platelet dysfunction
    (4) complete absorption when administered rectally

512. True statements regarding the use of opioids for pain management in children include

    (1) minor side effects occur more commonly in children than adults
    (2) the incidence of respiratory depression is directly related to dose
    (3) meperidine is preferred over morphine
    (4) tolerance is an uncommon clinical problem in children

513. True statements regarding the use of IV-PCA in children include

    (1) it is safe and effective
    (2) its use may be restricted by inability to activate the pump
    (3) it can be used in children age 7 and older
    (4) it is a universal therapy for postoperative pain control in children

514. Caudal block in children is

    (1) a widely used neural blockade technique
    (2) commonly performed in the lateral Sims position
    (3) performed as both single injection and continuous analgesia
    (4) an effective way to provide postoperative pain control

515. In a 4-year-old child scheduled for hypospadias repair, the advantages of combining a dorsal penile nerve block with general anesthesia over general anesthesia alone include

    (1) quick emergence
    (2) shorter recovery time
    (3) less requirement for inhalational anesthetics
    (4) decreased postoperative analgesic requirements

516. The nerves to be blocked in a fascia iliaca compartment block in a child include the

    (1) obturator nerve
    (2) lateral femoral cutaneous nerve
    (3) femoral nerve
    (4) sciatic nerve

517. After repair of an inguinal hernia in a child, infiltration analgesia of the surgical wound

    (1) produces analgesia comparable to that produced by a caudal technique
    (2) requires a local anesthetic dose equal to that of a caudal technique
    (3) results in lower local anesthetic concentrations in plasma compared with those in adults
    (4) is commonly used in neonates

518. True statements regarding pain assessment in nonverbal children include

    (1) neurophysiologic elements involved in pain perception are present in preterm infants
    (2) undesirable physiologic responses can be caused by pain in neonates
    (3) hormonal-metabolic responses to noxious stimuli are present in preterm infants
    (4) neonates experience pain

519. True statements regarding labor and the administration of regional anesthesia/analgesia include

    (1) epidural opioids produce a higher incidence of nausea in pregnant patients than in nonpregnant patients
    (2) cardiotoxicity from bupivacaine is more severe in pregnant patients than in nonpregnant patients
    (3) ephedrine is the preferred vasoconstrictor for use in pregnant patients
    (4) spinal opioids produce a lower incidence of pruritus in pregnant patients than in nonpregnant patients

520. Pain relief during the first stage of labor can be achieved by

    (1) lumbar sympathetic block
    (2) paracervical block
    (3) lumbar epidural block
    (4) pudendal nerve block

521. True statements regarding the administration of nitrous oxide (N_2O) for analgesia during labor include

    (1) no more than 50% N_2O in oxygen is recommended
    (2) accumulation occurs over time
    (3) elimination of the gas in the newborn takes hours
    (4) there are virtually no metabolites

522. Epidurally administered morphine as the sole analgesic during labor

    (1) has a delayed onset
    (2) has a low incidence of side effects
    (3) is inadequate for the second stage of labor
    (4) is comparable to epidural local anesthetic during the first stage of labor

523. Advantages of using 2-chloroprocaine administered epidurally to test for accidental intravenous injection include

    (1) no interference with subsequently administered opioids
    (2) rapid plasma hydrolysis
    (3) increased uterine blood flow
    (4) minimal fetal effects

524. An 85-year-old, 300-pound man underwent right upper lobectomy. Which of the following would be acceptable techniques to provide adequate postoperative pain relief?

    (1) Cryoneurolysis of the right intercostal nerves at multiple levels
    (2) Continuous segmental epidural analgesia with local anesthetic
    (3) Intercostal blocks with long-acting local anesthetic on the right at multiple levels
    (4) Intercostal blocks with long-acting local anesthetic bilaterally at multiple levels

525. Postoperative respiratory function tests that are more depressed after parenteral opioids than after epidural analgesia with opioids or local anesthetic include

    (1) peak expiratory flow rate
    (2) forced vital capacity
    (3) forced expiratory volume
    (4) functional residual capacity

PAIN MANAGEMENT

SUMMARY OF DIRECTIONS				
A	B	C	D	E
1,2,3 only	1,3 only	2,4 only	4 only	All are correct

526. Epidurally administered local anesthetics have which of the following effects on pain and the stress response?

    (1) T6–L2 blockade can abolish the stress response during lower abdominal surgery
    (2) There is inhibition of catecholamine discharge from the adrenal glands
    (3) Epidural blockade to the T5 sensory level is less effective in abolishing the stress response during upper abdominal than during lower abdominal surgery
    (4) There is a reduction in the negative nitrogen balance postoperatively

527. A 65-year-old man is about to undergo coronary artery bypass grafting. The administration of 1 mg/kg intravenous morphine prior to surgical incision will have which of the following effects on pain and the stress response?

    (1) Inhibition of ACTH release
    (2) Complete suppression of epinephrine release
    (3) Analgesia
    (4) Prevention of cortisol elevation

528. The stress response to acute injury and pain includes

    (1) increased renal and splanchnic blood flow
    (2) elevated levels of antidiuretic hormone
    (3) increased glomerular filtration
    (4) sodium and water retention

529. Which of the following medication regimens would be appropriate for use in a ventilated patient in an intensive care unit?

    (1) Intravenous morphine and diazepam
    (2) Epidural morphine and local anesthetic with intravenous diazepam
    (3) Intravenous fentanyl and midazolam
    (4) Epidural local anesthetic alone

530. Which of the following criteria can be used to support the diagnosis of brain death in the intensive care unit?

    (1) Light-fixed pupils
    (2) An isoelectric electroencephalogram recorded in part at full gain
    (3) No evidence of decerebrate or decorticate posturing or shivering
    (4) Heart rate increase of less than 5 beats per minute after intravenous atropine 0.04 mg/kg

531. A patient in the intensive care unit is in a persistent vegetative state and has total loss of cortical layers demonstrated on CT scan of the brain. The patient is able to breathe spontaneously. Which of the following interventions would be appropriate in the care of this patient?

    (1) New infusions of vasopressors to maintain hemodynamics
    (2) Mechanical ventilation if spontaneous respiration deteriorates
    (3) Insertion of an intraaortic balloon pump to augment cardiac function
    (4) Continued nutrition via a nasogastric tube

Pain Management in the Pediatric, Critical Care, and Obstetric Populations

Answers

506. The answer is C. *(Ferrante, p 488.)* Pain ratings can be reliably assessed using an analogue chromatic continuous scale (ACCS), which allows grading of a child's pain into a numeric value. The ACCS consists of a slide rule with graduated shades of red. The brightness of the color represents the intensity of pain. The child is asked to rate his or her pain by moving a sliding line indicator onto the appropriate color.

507. The answer is A. *(Bonica, p 1389.)* Maternal obstetric neuropathy after vaginal delivery is reported to occur in 1 in 2500 deliveries. The obturator, sciatic, or pudendal plexus can be injured by continuous pressure of the presenting part during labor or by forceps. The deficit is usually unilateral, but may be bilateral. One to two days after delivery, the patient may complain of burning, aching pain in the distribution of the injured nerve. There may be some motor impairment. The neuropathy is usually transient, and complete recovery often occurs after several weeks.

508. The answer is D. *(Ferrante, pp 487–488.)* Children between the ages of 2 and 7 years lack abstract thinking and the verbal skills necessary to express their feelings of pain. Therefore, nonverbal techniques are used to assess the intensity of their pain. A practical, reliable, and easy-to-apply bedside guide is a faces scale, such as the Oucher scale.

509. The answer is B. *(Capan, p 688.)* Spinal opioids can be effective analgesics in the postsurgical or trauma patient. They do not block the stress response during surgery. However, plasma glucose and cortisol levels are lower than the levels seen in patients who had general anesthesia and parenteral narcotics. Patients receiving epidural local anesthetics have even lower glucose and cortisol levels than patients receiving spinally administered narcotics. Spinal opioids do not have a significant effect on the pain pathways mediated by gamma-aminobutyric acid, nor on the sympathetic or proprioceptive afferents. Intraspinal and epidurally administered opioids block C-fiber nociceptive discharge preferentially.

510. The answer is D. *(Capan, p 687.)* Etomidate inhibits the activity of 17-α- and 11-β-hydroxylase, which catalyze the conversion of 11-deoxycortisol to active cortisol. It therefore inhibits cortisol production and has been implicated in increasing mortality in critically ill patients. Therefore, it is not recommended for use in the intensive care unit or in acute trauma patients.

511. The answer is A (1,2,3). *(Ferrante, p 490.)* Acetaminophen is widely used as an analgesic in children of all ages. It is not associated with Reye syndrome, as is aspirin. Other advantages over aspirin include lack of gastric irritation, lack of platelet dysfunction, and lack of cross-sensitivity to aspirin. Hypersensitivity is rare. A higher dose is recommended for rectal use (15 to 20 mg/kg). Absorption of acetaminophen is incomplete and unreliable when the drug is administered rectally.

512. **The answer is C (2,4).** (*Ferrante, pp 491–492.*) Meperidine is not routinely used in infants and children because of the prolonged elimination half-life in neonates (6 to 39 h) and because repeated administration may lead to an accumulation of the normeperidine metabolite, which may produce CNS excitation and seizures. The incidence of respiratory depression with mu agonists is directly related to the dose. Minor opioid side effects (e.g., nausea and vomiting) occur no more frequently in children than in adults. Tolerance is an uncommon clinical problem in children when opioids are used in appropriate doses for short periods of time.

513. **The answer is A (1,2,3).** (*Ferrante, pp 496–497.*) IV-PCA appears to be safe and effective in children and is frequently preferred by nursing staff, parents, and particularly adolescent patients. However, there are a small number of older children and adolescents who may not wish to be bothered with self-medication. They may feel indifferent and even dissatisfied with PCA and would rather receive analgesics by traditional methods. Therefore, PCA is not a universal therapy for postoperative pain control. IV-PCA can be used in children as young as 7 years of age. However, it may be restricted by age, developmental understanding of the purpose of PCA, and inability to activate the pump in the presence of muscular weakness or immobilization.

514. **The answer is E (all).** (*Ferrante, pp 496–501.*) Caudal anesthesia/analgesia is the most widely used neural blockade technique in children for the management of postoperative pain. Accumulating clinical experience suggests that caudal anesthesia/analgesia is simple to perform, reliable, and safe. The patient can be positioned in the lateral Sims position (preferred), prone, or in the knee-chest position. Single injections can be performed to augment a light general anesthetic, or a pediatric needle may be used to place an epidural catheter for continuous analgesia as well as postoperative pain control.

515. **The answer is E (all).** (*Ferrante, p 506.*) Dorsal penile nerve block (DPNB) is a reliable means of managing pain in children undergoing circumcision or correction of distal hypospadias. When DPNB is combined with general anesthesia for such procedures, there is a reduced requirement for inhalational anesthetics, quicker emergence, a shorter recovery time, and earlier discharge from the hospital compared with the administration of general anesthesia alone. Postoperative analgesic requirements are also diminished for a considerable period of time when long-acting local anesthetics are used.

516. **The answer is A (1,2,3).** (*Ferrante, p 510.*) The fascia iliaca compartment block is a relatively new technique whereby femoral, lateral femoral cutaneous, and obturator neural blockade can be accomplished with a single injection. These nerves lie on the anterior surface of the iliac muscle and are enclosed by iliac fascia. The iliac compartment is safely approached at the junction of the lateral one-third and medial two-thirds of the inguinal ligament.

517. **The answer is B (1,3).** (*Ferrante, p 512.*) In children, injection of local anesthetic into the incision at the end of inguinal herniotomy produces analgesia comparable to that rendered by caudal analgesia. Doses of 0.5 mL/kg of 0.25% bupivacaine are effective for wound infiltration and are half the dose required for caudal blockade (1 mL/kg). The absorption of bupivacaine from subcutaneous infiltration is considerably slower in children than adults, and the resultant plasma concentrations of local anesthetic are far below toxic levels. Unfortunately, infiltration analgesia is widely underused or not used at all in neonates undergoing surgery.

518. **The answer is E (all).** (*Ferrante, pp 486–487.*) Available data indicate that the neurophysiologic and neurochemical components necessary for the transduction, transmission, modulation, and perception of nociception are present in term and preterm infants. The hormonal-metabolic responses to noxious stimuli are also intact. Similarly, undesirable physiologic responses can be provoked by pain. Term and preterm infants can undergo substantial changes in hemodynamics, oxygen saturation, and intracranial pressure in response to noxious surgical stimuli. Thus, in contrast to previously held beliefs, the evidence suggests that neonates experience pain and should be treated for it.

519. The answer is A (1,2,3). (*Raj, p 392.*) Cardiotoxicity from bupivacaine is more severe during pregnancy, and its treatment is more difficult. Epidural and spinal opioid therapy produces a higher incidence of nausea and pruritus in pregnant women. It is also associated with activation of herpes simplex labialis, which may raise concerns regarding newborn infection. Should a vasopressor be required, ephedrine is preferred, since it has the least detrimental effect on uterine perfusion.

520. The answer is A (1,2,3). (*Raj, pp 393–395.*) Pain relief during the first stage of labor can be achieved by local anesthetic injection near paracervical and lumbar sympathetic fibers as well as by lumbar epidural or spinal blocks. The pain of the first stage of labor is visceral in origin, emanating from stretching and distention of the cervix and lower uterine segment and referred to lumbar and lower thoracic dermatomes. A pudendal nerve block is helpful during the second stage of labor when pain originates from perineal structures and is primarily transmitted via sacral afferent fibers.

521. The answer is D (4). (*Raj, p 395.*) Nitrous oxide analgesia is commonly used in obstetric patients when regional analgesia is not available or is unwanted. Typically, the patient self-administers the anesthetic using an approved apparatus that delivers no more than 70% nitrous oxide in oxygen through a face mask or mouthpiece. The physical properties of nitrous oxide are such that accumulation over time is negligible and elimination of the gas in the newborn is virtually completed within a few minutes of birth. The elimination pathway is via the lungs. There are no clinically significant metabolites.

522. The answer is B (1,3). (*Raj, p 396.*) In general, epidural opioids as sole analgesics during labor have shown disappointing results. Epidural morphine, when administered alone, requires larger dosing. The onset of analgesia is delayed and is not comparable to that produced by epidural local anesthetics during the first stage of labor. Epidural morphine used alone is inadequate during the second stage of labor. The incidence of bothersome side effects from epidural morphine is high when compared with more lipid-soluble agents.

523. The answer is C (2,4). (*Raj, p 402.*) An alternative to epinephrine when testing for accidental epidural intravenous administration of solution is the use of 2-chloroprocaine. Advantages of 2-chloroprocaine include rapid plasma hydrolysis, which minimizes systemic or fetal effects, and lack of effect on uterine blood flow. Advantages of lidocaine include lack of deleterious effect on the potency of subsequently injected bupivacaine or opioids (unlike 2-chloroprocaine, which interferes with both) and more prolonged analgesia when injected in the epidural space.

524. The answer is A (1,2,3). (*Capan, p 691.*) In elderly patients with high body mass indices, bilateral intercostal nerve blocks at T5–T11 were found to change the relationship between closing capacity and functional residual capacity, leading to hypoxemia and hypercarbia. This did not occur in younger patients with normal body mass indices. Cryoneurolysis, unilateral intercostal nerve blocks, and epidural analgesia are acceptable techniques for providing postoperative analgesia and decreasing pulmonary dysfunction.

525. The answer is E (all). (*Capan, p 690.*) Postoperatively, peak expiratory flow rate, forced vital capacity, forced expiratory volume, and functional residual capacity are all reduced more when parenteral opioids are used than when epidural analgesia using either local anesthetics or opioids is used. Splinting and depressed respiratory function due to inadequate analgesia result in a lowering of the arterial oxygen, less efficient coughing, deep breathing, and removal of bronchial secretions, which may predispose patients to atelectasis and pulmonary infection.

526. The answer is E (all). *(Capan, p 688.)* Neural blockade with local anesthetics abolishes the pain and stress response by blocking the somatic and sympathetic afferent pathways. T6–L2 blockade successfully abolishes the stress response to lower abdominal surgery but is not as effective (even with T9 blockade) in upper abdominal surgery. There is a reduction in the total negative nitrogen balance during the first 4 postoperative days if epidural analgesia with local anesthetic is given for the first 24 h postoperatively. In general, there are also reduced plasma glucose and cortisol levels. However, it does not ablate the moderate rise in serum cortisol seen immediately after the surgical incision.

527. The answer is B (1,3). *(Capan, p 687.)* Intravenous administration of 1 mg/kg morphine has been shown to inhibit ACTH release and suppress the pituitary-adrenal axis, but it cannot suppress the rise in plasma catecholamines during cardiac surgery. Higher doses of opioid can partially suppress the endocrine-metabolic response until bypass, after which marked elevations of cortisol, epinephrine, norepinephrine, and antidiuretic hormone occur. Inhibition of the stress response requires significantly higher doses than those required to obtain analgesia.

528. The answer is C (2,4). *(Capan, p 686.)* The stress response to acute injury and pain results in increased sympathetic efferent activity and elevated serum levels of epinephrine, norepinephrine, growth hormone, cortisol, renin, aldosterone, antidiuretic hormone, enkephalins, and endorphins. Tachycardia, hypertension, decreased renal and splanchnic blood flow, decreased glomerular filtration, hyperglycemia, and sodium and water retention occur. Initially, the stress response may serve as an important mechanism to preserve vital functions. Once treatment has begun, a continued stress response can be deleterious to the patient who is likely to be at risk for end-organ ischemia or infarction.

529. The answer is A (1,2,3). *(Shoemaker, pp 796–799.)* Ventilated patients in an intensive care setting require analgesia as well as sedation to alleviate anxiety and promote sleep. Intravenous opioids and benzodiazepines administered by infusion and supplemented with boluses as needed are quite effective. Epidural analgesia should be supplemented with intravenous benzodiazepines or other sedating medications that will provide anxiolysis and promote sleep.

530. The answer is E (all). *(Shoemaker, pp 968–969.)* The definition of brain death is the permanent loss of all integrated brain functions. The patient is not experiencing pain or suffering. As such, it is extremely important to elimate all medications and correct hemodynamic variables that may be contributing to the comatose condition before one declares the patient brain dead. The patient should have adequate blood pressure and temperature above 34°C (93.2°F) and be free of alcohol, toxins, and medications that could depress brain function. A detailed and thoroughly documented clinical examination should be performed and then repeated no sooner than 2 h after the initial examination. Body temperature, blood ethanol level, and toxicology screens should be documented. In the absence of muscle relaxants, there should be no spontaneous movement and no evidence of decerebrate or decorticate posturing or shivering and there should be no spontaneous breathing for 3 min (at $Paco_2$ > 60 torr at the end of the test). If the patient has pulmonary disease, the Pao_2 must be less than 50 torr at the end of the test. The patient must have light-fixed pupils and the absence of corneal reflexes, response to painful stimuli, response to upper and lower airway stimulation, ocular response to head turning, and ocular response to ear irrigation with 50 mL of ice water. Intravenous atropine 0.04 mg/kg should fail to increase the heart rate by more than 5 beats per minute. An isoelectric electroencephalogram recorded in part at full gain should also be obtained. The ultimate criterion of brain death is the complete absence of cerebral blood flow, which can be documented by bilateral internal carotid and vertebral arteriography or by radionuclide cerebral imaging.

531. The answer is D (4). (*Shoemaker, pp 969–972.*) A patient who is not brain dead but has permanently lost consciousness can be described as one whose personality, memory, interaction with others, and emotional states are gone, but whose physical vegetative functions and reflexes persist. If cerebral arteriography and modified CT scanning of the brain demonstrate total loss of cortical layers, the irreversibility of the patient's unconscious state can be verified. At that point, it is justifiable to proceed on the premise that life-sustaining therapies will no longer benefit the patient and are therefore not indicated. A patient on a ventilator may be weaned in spite of deteriorating vital signs and blood gases. Even nutrition may be withheld, though commonly it will be continued while new therapies, ventilation, antibiotics, and pressor support are withheld.

Psychological Aspects of Pain

DIRECTIONS: Each question below contains suggested responses. Select the **one best** response.

532. Which of the following statements regarding suicide is true?

    (A) Less than 10 percent of patients who commit suicide have seen their physicians in the last 3 months
    (B) Women between the ages of 40 and 50 have the highest suicide rate
    (C) Five percent of suicide victims use medications prescribed by their physicians to commit suicide
    (D) Depressed chronic pain patients should routinely be asked about suicidal ideation

533. All the following statements regarding conversion disorder are true EXCEPT

    (A) an alteration in physical functioning occurs as a consequence of psychological conflict
    (B) the patient is conscious of the connection between the physical dysfunction and the psychological stress at the time it occurs
    (C) limb paralysis and blindness can be symptoms of conversion disorder
    (D) pain is the most common conversion symptom encountered clinically

534. All the following are psychological stages that a patient with a terminal disease will typically experience EXCEPT

    (A) anger
    (B) transference
    (C) bargaining
    (D) acceptance
    (E) denial

535. A 30-year-old woman complains of abdominal pain that began at age 8. Multiple medical and surgical evaluations have been completely within normal limits. The patient states that she has "always been sickly" and that her mother "had the same problem." There is no history of childhood trauma or abuse. She has been unable to work for the last 4 years. Which of the following psychological diagnoses best describes her condition?

    (A) Somatization disorder
    (B) Conversion disorder
    (C) Hypochondriasis
    (D) Major depression

536. Which three scales of the Minnesota Multiphasic Personality Inventory (MMPI) compose the "conversion V" frequently seen in chronic pain patients?

    (A) Paranoia, hysteria, depression
    (B) Hypochondriasis, psychasthenia, depression
    (C) Social introversion, depression, hysteria
    (D) Hypochondriasis, depression, hysteria

537. The cluster of psychological effects characteristic of patients suffering from prolonged chronic pain is called

    (A) psychosomatic illness
    (B) abnormal illness behavior
    (C) malingering
    (D) conversion reaction

538. The most frequent affective problem seen with acute pain is

    (A) depression
    (B) anger
    (C) anxiety
    (D) panic

539. Which of the following statements is true regarding anxiety and its effect on pain perception?

    (A) Anxiety does not amplify the intensity of a painful stimulus
    (B) Patients with a high degree of trait anxiety have the same degree of pre- and postsurgical situational anxiety as patients with low trait anxiety
    (C) Patients with chronic anxiety disorder or panic disorder have a similar incidence of emergency room visits for pain complaints as patients without those disorders
    (D) Anxiety can result from the anticipation or presence of uncontrolled pain

540. All the following statements regarding relaxation training are true EXCEPT

    (A) it has not been helpful in patients with chronic abdominal pain
    (B) it has been helpful in patients with headaches, temporomandibular joint (TMJ) dysfunction, arthritis, and myocardial infarction
    (C) progressive muscle relaxation, proper breathing, and dissociative visualization are phases of the integrative approach to relaxation training
    (D) it induces a low level of arousal, which may be adversive in some patients
    (E) myoclonic jerks, cramping, muscle soreness, transient respiratory difficulties, and dissociation have occurred

541. Psychological aids in the management of headache pain include all the following EXCEPT

    (A) relaxation training
    (B) electroconvulsive therapy (ECT)
    (C) biofeedback training
    (D) operant pain control techniques
    (E) cognitive therapy

542. Operant conditioning and reinforcement of chronic pain behaviors occur in which of the following situations?

    (A) Around-the-clock administration of oral opioids
    (B) "Working through the pain" to complete activities of daily living without assistance
    (C) Solicitous attention from a helpful spouse with encouragement to rest or "take it easy"
    (D) Modification of the work and home environment to encourage full participation in usual activities

543. The term *malingering* may be used to describe all the following situations EXCEPT

    (A) willful fabrication of symptoms and signs
    (B) unconscious ascription of pain to a cause associated with potential gain
    (C) continuing complaint of disability after the physical cause has ceased to exist
    (D) magnification of symptoms and signs

544. Which of the following statements is true regarding biofeedback?

(A) It is more effective in treatment of chronic pain than is relaxation training
(B) Equipment and technological support are required to perform biofeedback
(C) EMG feedback cannot be used to treat muscle tension headaches
(D) Thermal biofeedback has reversed diabetic neuropathy
(E) There is no role for biofeedback in the treatment of phantom limb pain

545. A 69-year-old woman with breast cancer and multiple bony metastases complains of her slowly increasing requirement of intrathecal morphine and the consequent increase in the nausea associated with the increased dose. Work-up by the oncology team did not reveal further progression of the disease. What is the best explanation for this patient's predicament?

(A) She is addicted to the drug and keeps wanting a higher dose
(B) The catheter is no longer in the intrathecal space
(C) She is physically dependent on the drug and is nauseated because she is going through withdrawal
(D) She is developing tolerance to the analgesic effects of intrathecal morphine

DIRECTIONS: Each question below contains four suggested responses of which **one or more** is correct. Select

A	if	**1, 2, and 3**	are correct
B	if	**1 and 3**	are correct
C	if	**2 and 4**	are correct
D	if	**4**	is correct
E	if	**1, 2, 3, and 4**	are correct

546. Symptoms that are typical of patients with multiple personality disorder (MPD) that are also found in chronic pain patients include

    (1) neurologic complaints such as seizures, numbness and tingling, motor weakness, and functional limb paralysis
    (2) GI complaints such as unexplained nausea and irritable bowel syndrome
    (3) reproduction system complaints such as pelvic pain and dysmenorrhea
    (4) migraine-like headaches

547. The multidimensional concept of acute pain consists of which of the following factors?

    (1) The sensory-discriminative aspect of pain
    (2) The motivational-emotional dimension of pain
    (3) The social-cultural dimension of pain
    (4) The conceptual-judgmental dimension of pain

548. True statements describing the effect of cognitive and behavioral factors on pain perception include

    (1) selective attention has been shown to decrease the psychologic response to painful stimuli
    (2) operant learning can lead to habitual pain behavior
    (3) seeing someone else go through the painful experience in a calm, controlled manner increases the patient's ability to undergo the procedure with less discomfort
    (4) preprocedural instruction has no effect on the quality of pain experienced

549. True statements regarding the psychophysiologic response to acute pain include which of the following?

    (1) Acute pain is an emotionally neutral experience
    (2) The release of norepinephrine at sympathetic nerve endings can directly activate nociceptors
    (3) Reflex skeletal muscle tension decreases activation of muscle nociceptors
    (4) Relaxation and mental distraction decrease the aversive qualities of acute pain

Psychological Aspects of Pain

Answers

532. The answer is D. (*Bonica, p 318.*) Elderly males with a chronic illness have the highest risk of suicide. Eighty percent of patients who commit suicide have seen their physician in the last 3 months, and 50 percent of them commit suicide with medications prescribed by a physician. All depressed patients should be routinely asked about suicidal thoughts. If patients answer "yes" to questions about having thoughts of harming themselves, it is important to pursue further risk assessment before discharging them from your immediate care.

533. The answer is B. (*Bonica, pp 301–302.*) Conversion disorder is the loss or alteration of physical functioning that is temporarily associated with a psychosocial stressor. The patient is not conscious of intentionally producing the physical symptom in response to the psychic stressor. Paralysis and blindness are often described as classic symptoms of conversion disorder. However, pain is the most common conversion symptom encountered clinically. Sexual dysfunction is also common.

534. The answer is B. (*Raj, p 74.*) The distinguishing characteristic of terminal pain is the psychological impact of impending death. This may be divided into five stages: denial, anger, bargaining, depression, and acceptance.

535. The answer is A. (*Bonica, pp 301–303.*) The patient has a somatization disorder (also called *hysteria* or *Briquet's syndrome*). Patients often present with a long history of physical complaints before 30 years of age. Many have undergone comprehensive medical evaluations and surgical interventions without diagnosis of any significant disease process. They also have impaired social development because of their perceived illness. Occupational development is also affected. Many do not work or work at jobs limited by their perceived pain.

In conversion disorder, there is loss of a physical function that is temporally related to a psychosocial stressor. Sexual dysfunction, pain, blindness, and paralysis have been described as manifestations of the psychological conflict experienced by patients with conversion disorder.

Hypochondriasis is the excessive preoccupation with disease and with one's health. Hypochondriacs believe that a disease process exists despite medical evaluation and reassurance over long periods of time. Patients may pay obsessive attention to perceived pain symptoms without significant fear or depression. They complain to family and physicians and are not reassured by normal medical examinations and tests results.

536. The answer is D. (*Bonica, p 193.*) Many patients with prolonged chronic pain have elevation of the hypochondriasis, depression, and hysteria scores of 2 or more standard deviations above the mean. This is considered clinically significant. Patients with acute pain frequently have slightly elevated hypochondriasis, depression, and hysteria scores, but not to a clinically significant degree. Once the pain resolves, the mild elevation returns closer to or within the normal range.

537. The answer is B. (*Bonica, p 192.*) Abnormal illness behavior consists of reactive depression, hypochondriasis, somatic preoccupation, disease conviction, and a tendency to deny life problems unrelated to the painful physical problem. It is characteristic of patients suffering from prolonged chronic pain. Psychosomatic illness, malingering, and conversion reaction may occur, but are not consistent characteristics of prolonged chronic pain.

538. The answer is C. (*Bonica, p 124.*) Apprehension with heightened autonomic arousal (anxiety) is the most common negative emotional response seen in the setting of acute pain. Other emotional disorders such as depression, anger, panic, dissociative or *chronic* anxiety behaviors may complicate the assessment of acute pain problems. They are usually due to underlying problems that preceded the acute pain state.

539. The answer is D. (*Bonica, pp 124–125.*) Anxiety can be defined as apprehension or fear occurring in conjunction with patterns of heightened autonomic arousal. Pain perception may be intensified by anxiety related to the anticipation or experience of uncontrolled pain and by the presence of interpersonal conflict, conditioning, or chronic anxiety disorder. Patients who have a predisposition to respond to situations perceived as threatening with apprehension and heightened autonomic response are described as having *trait* anxiety. Patients with a high degree of trait anxiety have much higher pre- and postsurgical situational anxiety than patients with low trait anxiety. Patients with anxiety or panic disorders have a significantly higher incidence of presentation to the emergency room with pain complaints, especially chest pain.

540. The answer is A. (*Tollison, pp 178–182.*) Relaxation training has been successful as adjunctive treatment of tension headaches, migraine, posttraumatic headaches, lower back pain, TMJ pain, myofascial pain, arthritis, dysmenorrhea, cancer pain, phantom pain, and abdominal pain. The integrative approach to relaxation training incorporates the successfully used techniques of progressive muscle relaxation, proper breathing, and dissociative visualization. Some patients have adverse reactions to the state of low arousal, so that relaxing techniques should be modified to include high-arousal imagery, such as mountain climbing or sky diving, during dissociative visualization. The relaxation response may lower blood pressure and normalize elevated blood sugar and thyroid function; therefore, patients on antihypertensive medications, antidiabetic medications, or thyroid medications should be carefully monitored and have medications adjusted as appropriate.

541. The answer is B. (*Tollison, pp 264–272.*) Relaxation training is especially helpful in treatment of muscle contraction or tension headaches. Thermal biofeedback is helpful in managing migraines and combined vascular and muscular contraction headaches. Frontal EMG biofeedback has been helpful in muscle contraction headaches. Cognitive therapy focuses on improving the patient's problem-solving abilities, improving coping skills, and decreasing the stressors that may cause headaches. This is especially useful in patients with muscle contraction headaches. Operant pain control techniques, which include extinction of pain behaviors and reinforcement of nonpain behaviors, have been successful in the treatment of some migraine patients and patients with psychogenic headaches. ECT has not been used to treat headaches.

542. The answer is C. (*Bonica, pp 295–296.*) Behavior that has positive or reinforcing consequences tends to persist in chronic pain patients. When an injury or disease has elicited pain behaviors, conditioning may occur if there is frequent reinforcement of the pain behavior. This will make it difficult for the patient to decrease the pain behavior and participate more actively in recovery. Reinforcement of pain behavior may occur when the patient receives special attention, gets permission to rest, or takes medications that may have pleasurable side effects, such as mild euphoria or anxiolysis, on an "as needed" basis. If the chronic pain patient is "coddled" by a solicitous spouse who allows the patient freedom from normal household responsibilities, this will also reinforce pain behavior.

543. The answer is B. (*Tollison, p 337.*) Malingering can be defined as the conscious alteration of health for gain. Malingering can manifest itself in a variety of ways. There may be (1) pretension, in which no physical illness exists and the patient willfully fabricates symptoms and signs; (2) exaggeration, in which symptoms and signs are magnified; (3) perseveration, which is a continuing complaint after the physical cause of the disability has ceased to exist; or (4) allegation, in which a true disability is present, but the patient fraudulently ascribes it to a cause associated with potential gain.

544. The answer is B. (*Tollison, pp 178–179.*) Biofeedback has been used to treat muscle tension headaches, migraine, cluster headaches, posttraumatic headaches, lower back pain, arthritis, TMJ pain, myofascial pain, phantom pain, benign chest pain, angina, dysmenorrhea, postherpetic neuralgia, causalgia, sickle cell disease, and burn pain. Three commonly used forms of biofeedback are EMG biofeedback to decrease muscle tension, thermal feedback to increase finger temperature, and cephalic blood volume pulse feedback at the cephalic temporal artery. The scientific basis for the use of biofeedback in the treatment of pain has not been fully elucidated.

545. The answer is D (4). (*Bonica, p 1969.*) The patient is most likely developing tolerance to the analgesic effects of the intrathecal morphine while continuing to complain of the adverse side effect of nausea as the intrathecal dose is increased. The mechanism by which tolerance develops is not known. The development of tolerance can be minimized by selecting the lowest effective narcotic dose; placing the catheter as close as possible to the cord level of the painful areas; giving multiple, small, divided doses rather than one or two large, daily boluses; and using low-dose continuous infusions whenever possible.

546. The answer is E (all). (*Livengood, Pain Digest 4:191–194, 1994.*) The pain complaints and somatoform symptoms typical of chronic pain patients are often present in patients with multiple personality disorder (MPD). Multiple personality disorder is a severe, chronic dissociative disorder in which two or more distinct personalities or personality states exist within the same person and recurrently take control of the person's behavior. The switching of personalities is often covert and subtle. Patients with MPD have significantly more somatic complaints than other patients with psychiatric illness. Analgesic medication or other treatment modalities for pain control may not be effective unless the disorder is treated.

547. The answer is E (all). (*Bonica, p 124.*) The multidimensional conceptualization of pain describes the complex interaction of many factors, such as the motivational-emotional, social-cultural, and conceptual-judgmental dimensions specific to each individual in response to noxious sensory input. The model below illustrates how each component of the pain experience can affect the others.

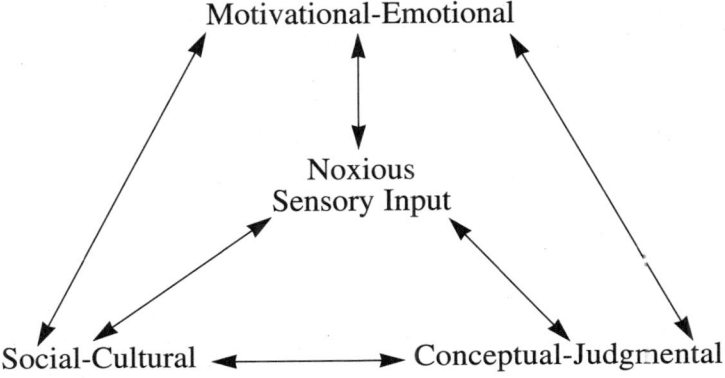

For example, a patient who is anxious prior to surgery will experience more pain than a nonanxious patient. However, if the patient is undergoing an elective procedure, is not overly concerned about the outcome of the procedure (e.g., no fear of cancer), or comes from a stoical culture, the conceptual and cultural dimensions underlying the pain experience will likely decrease the patient's reaction to a noxious stimulus.

548. The answer is A (1,2,3). *(Bonica, pp 125–127.)* Selective attention can decrease or prevent pain perception. Psychological techniques of pain control, such as hypnosis, may be successful because of diversion of attention away from the painful stimuli. Learning processes, such as operant learning, instructional learning, and social learning (modeling), have a significant effect on the quality and intensity of the pain experienced. Operant learning is characterized by behaviors that recur because of rewards that follow those behaviors. For example, if pain behavior results in solicitude and increased attention from a spouse, the pain behavior is rewarded. As such, it may become habitual and can be defined as operant learning if it occurs outside the awareness of the person. Social learning (modeling) is learning by imitation. Patients may learn to respond to painful stimuli with specific behaviors they have seen from others. For example, children who have observed other children in the dental chair responding in a calm, controlled manner are more likely to respond in a similar way. Instructional learning, such as review of the painful procedure and sensations that may be experienced, allows the patient to develop cognitive defense mechanisms that increase the ability to cope with the stress and anxiety associated with painful stimuli.

549. The answer is C (2,4). *(Bonica, pp 122–123.)* Response to acute pain involves both emotional and physical components. Emotional distress increases sympathetic activity, which causes release of norepinephrine at sympathetic nerve endings. Norepinephrine directly activates tissue nociceptors. Skeletal muscle spasm, which is increased by anxiety, activates muscle nociceptors. Relaxation and mental distraction can decrease the emotional response to acute pain and thereby lessen activation of peripheral nociceptors.

Compensation, Disability Assessment, and Medicolegal Issues

DIRECTIONS: Each question below contains suggested responses. Select the **one best** response.

550. Which of the following drugs is a schedule I substance?

    (A) Nalorphine
    (B) Hydromorphone
    (C) Heroin
    (D) Diazepam

551. Under the Controlled Substances Act, which of the following drug schedules is thought to have the highest potential for abuse?

    (A) Schedule II
    (B) Schedule III
    (C) Schedule IV
    (D) Schedule V

552. All the following statements regarding the Controlled Substances Act (CSA) are true EXCEPT

    (A) controlled substances may be prescribed for a legitimate medical purpose not indicated in the approved labeling
    (B) dronabinol (synthetic tetrahydrocannabinol) may be prescribed for treatment of nausea and vomiting in patients with chronic, nonmalignant pain
    (C) the CSA limits the number of refills per prescription, but does not limit the amount or duration of use
    (D) physicians may use opioid analgesics to treat intractable chronic pain in patients with a current or prior history of drug abuse

553. All the following are important components of evaluation of a low back impairment EXCEPT

    (A) EMG and radiologic studies
    (B) general medical examination, including assessment of joint mobility, muscle strength, and sensory abnormalities
    (C) lie detector test
    (D) a "whole-man impairment" rating

554. A concert pianist and a vice president of a major corporation have both suffered the loss of the second finger of the dominant hand. Which of the following statements is true regarding the condition of impairment or disability due to the injury?

    (A) The concert pianist is more impaired than the vice president
    (B) The concert pianist and vice president are equally disabled
    (C) The concert pianist and vice president are both handicapped
    (D) The concert pianist is more disabled than the vice president
    (E) The concert pianist is more handicapped than the vice president

555. Disability is correctly characterized by which of the following?

(A) It is a condition that relates to function relative to work or other obligations
(B) It is a condition that relates to the effects of a disease process or injury
(C) It is a condition that requires the use of an assistive device to perform activities of daily living
(D) It is expressed as a percentage of the body as a whole
(E) It is a term that can be used interchangeably with the term *handicap*

COMPENSATION, DISABILITY ASSESSMENT, AND MEDICOLEGAL ISSUES

DIRECTIONS: Each question below contains four suggested responses of which **one or more** is correct. Select

A	if	**1, 2, and 3**	are correct
B	if	**1 and 3**	are correct
C	if	**2 and 4**	are correct
D	if	**4**	is correct
E	if	**1, 2, 3, and 4**	are correct

556. True statements regarding the Controlled Substances Act (CSA) include which of the following?
   (1) A physician may register to detoxify or maintain narcotic-addicted patients using long-acting narcotics (e.g., methadone, levorphanol, or MS-Contin)
   (2) An *addict* is defined as someone who uses a narcotic drug so as to endanger public health or safety, or who has lost control over narcotic use
   (3) A physician may not use opioids to treat chronic intractable pain in patients who have a current history of drug abuse
   (4) A physician may maintain or detoxify a patient on chronic opioids prescribed to treat medical or surgical conditions, including pain

557. True statements regarding confidentiality of medical records include which of the following?
   (1) The payer of worker's compensation claims has rights to all records upon request
   (2) Any agent acting on behalf of the Health Care Finance Administration (Medicare) may have access at any time to medical records of patients reimbursed by the Administration
   (3) Private indemnity insurance companies must obtain express written consent from the patient prior to reviewing the medical record
   (4) Release of mental health records may require special consent even though they are integrated into the general medical record

558. True statements regarding worker's compensation include
   (1) medical expenses are paid
   (2) there is monetary compensation for pain and suffering
   (3) there is compensation for lost wages
   (4) fault or negligence of the employer must be established

559. The Social Security Administration uses a number of criteria for determination of eligibility for disability benefits. The sequential evaluation for determination of benefits includes which of the following factors?
   (1) Age
   (2) Educational background
   (3) Previous work history
   (4) Residual functional capacity

560. Sedentary work is characterized by which of the following criteria?
   (1) Lifting a maximum of 10 lb
   (2) Pushing and pulling of arm or leg controls
   (3) Requirement of occasional walking and standing, but mostly sitting
   (4) Carrying objects weighing up to 10 lb

561. Criteria for good documentation in a medical record include
   (1) objective information
   (2) time-specific charting
   (3) legible writing
   (4) use of only approved abbreviations

SUMMARY OF DIRECTIONS				
A	B	C	D	E
1,2,3 only	1,3 only	2,4 only	4 only	All are correct

562. Requirements for informed consent include statements of

   (1) material risks
   (2) expected outcome
   (3) alternative treatments
   (4) effects of no treatment

563. The term *handicap*

   (1) applies to a person who has impairment that substantially limits life's activities
   (2) is related to but different from the term *impairment*
   (3) can be applied to an impaired person who requires the use of an assistive device to perform activities of daily living
   (4) can be applied to a disabled person who requires modification of the environment to perform activities of daily living

564. Impairment may be defined as

   (1) a condition that relates to a disease process
   (2) a condition that relates to function relative to work or other obligations
   (3) derangement or loss of use of any body part, system, or function
   (4) the limiting, loss, or absence of the capacity of a person to meet personal, social, or occupational demands

Compensation, Disability Assessment, and Medicolegal Issues

Answers

550. The answer is C. *("Guidelines," Federation Bulletin 67:47–50, 1980.)* The Controlled Substances Act has divided drugs under its jurisdiction into five schedules. Schedule I drugs have a high potential for abuse and no accepted medical use in the United States. Examples of schedule I drugs include heroin, marijuana, LSD, psilocybin, and methaqualone.

551. The answer is A. *("Guidelines," Federation Bulletin 67:47–50, 1980.)* Schedule II drugs have a high potential for abuse and a high rate of psychological or physical dependence. Narcotic analgesics are schedule II drugs. Nonnarcotic drugs such as amphetamines, methylphenidate, and pentobarbital are also schedule II.

Schedule IV drugs are thought to have less potential for abuse than schedule I, II, and III drugs. Examples of schedule IV drugs are benzodiazepines, phenobarbital, meprobamate, chloral hydrate, and dextropropoxyphene (Darvon).

Schedule V drugs have the lowest potential for abuse of the drugs under the jurisdiction of the Controlled Substances Act. Antitussives and antidiarrheal preparations that contain narcotics in limited quantities are schedule V drugs.

552. The answer is B. *(Joranson, Federation Bulletin 79:15–49, 1992.)* Use of dronabinol is strictly limited to patients suffering from nausea and vomiting due to cancer chemotherapy. While the CSA allows controlled substances to be prescribed for legitimate off-label purposes, a specific exception to this rule has been made for dronabinol. Off-label prescription of dronabinol exposes the physician to the risk of criminal and civil action.

553. The answer is C. *(Bonica, pp 641–646.)* Impairment is defined by the World Health Organization (WHO) as "the loss or functional limitation of an organ or system of the body or the mind which is stable after maximum rehabilitation and nonprogressive at the time of evaluation." The AMA *Guides to the Evaluation of Permanent Impairment* is useful in quantifying the level of impairment in chronic pain patients. Using the AMA guidelines, an evaluation of impairment must include a general medical examination and functional assessment. Relevant EMG and radiologic studies must be obtained. Correlation with physical findings should be attempted. The AMA guidelines provide tables that translate multiple impairments of body parts into a "whole-man impairment rating." Maximum impairment due to back dysfunction is 60 percent of the whole-man impairment.

Disability is different from impairment. Disability is defined by the World Health Organization as "task-specific limitation of performance." A person is handicapped if "the disabled status creates a socioeconomic disadvantage."

554. The answer is D. *(AMA Guides to the Evaluation of Permanent Impairment, pp 1–2.)* Both the concert pianist and the company vice president have an impairment due to the loss of their digit. However, the concert pianist is significantly more disabled because the pianist will not be able to perform but the vice president will still be able to do the job. They are not significantly handicapped because they can still perform life's activities without the use of assistive devices or modification of the environment.

555. The answer is A. *(AMA Guides to the Evaluation of Permanent Impairment, pp 1–2.)* Disability is the limiting, loss, or absence of the capacity of a person to meet personal, social, or occupational demands, or to meet statutory or regulatory requirements. Disability relates to function relative to work or other obligations and activities of daily living. It may be characterized as temporary, permanent, partial, or total. Methods of assessing functional performance include measurement of range of motion, strength, endurance, and work simulation. *Disability* is not synonymous with *handicap*. When an impairment is associated with an obstacle to useful activity, a handicap may exist; assistive devices or modifications of the environment are often required to accomplish life's basic activities.

556. The answer is C (2,4). *(Joranson, Federation Bulletin 79:15–49, 1992.)* The CSA defines an addict as someone who uses a narcotic drug so as to endanger public health or safety, or who has lost control over narcotic use. The CSA makes a very clear distinction between the use of opioids to treat chronic medical conditions and the use of opioids to treat opioid addiction. Prescribing opioids to maintain a narcotic addiction is not considered a legitimate use. A physician must register with the federal government prior to prescribing narcotics as treatment of addiction. Only methadone may be prescribed for treatment of addiction. A physician may prescribe opioid analgesics as treatment for intractable pain in patients with a current or prior history of drug abuse.

557. The answer is E (all). *(Anastasio, J Am Med Rec Assoc 61:52–61, 1990. Griffith, Med Staff Couns 5:31–37, 1991.)* Worker's compensation claimants must allow access to medical records any time they are requested by the payee. Medicare agents also have access to medical records of any patient receiving Medicare benefits. Private insurers must ask the permission of the patient to view the medical records. Mental health records, even though they may be part of the medical record, may not be released without the specific consent of the patient in many states. It is important to clarify what laws are in effect regarding mental health records in your particular state. If specific consent is required, unauthorized release of mental health records may result in damages against the clinic or physician involved.

558. The answer is B (1,3). *(Tollison, p 644.)* Worker's compensation provides injured workers with funds to cover medical expenses and lost wages. It does not, however, totally replace lost income. A totally disabled worker will receive approximately two-thirds of his average weekly wage. There is no compensation for pain and suffering, nor is there any determination of fault or negligence on the part of the employer or the worker.

559. The answer is E (all). *(Tollison, pp 635–636.)* To determine eligibility for Social Security funds, the applicant must undergo a sequential evaluation process that considers the applicant's ability to perform work despite any functional restrictions associated with physical impairment. Medical and psychological variables are considered, along with the applicant's age, educational background, and previous work history. The applicant must undergo a medical evaluation to determine residual functional capacity. Both exertional factors (evaluation of the applicant's ability to perform work functions in several different work environments) and nonexertional factors (evaluation of the applicant's cognitive capabilities) are part of the evaluation of residual functional capacity.

560. The answer is B (1,3). *(Tollison, p 639.)* *Sedentary work* is defined as lifting 10 lb maximum, with occasional lifting or carrying of small, light objects. The work involves mostly sitting, with a small amount of walking or standing to perform job duties.

To perform *light work*, the employee must be able to lift up to 20 lb and carry up to 10 lb. Walking or standing may be required for significant periods of the work day. Pushing or pulling of arm or leg controls in the sitting or standing position is also classified as light work.

For *medium work*, the employee must be able to lift 50 lb frequently and carry up to 25 lb.

For *heavy work*, the employee must be able to lift up to 100 lb frequently and carry up to 50 lb.

For *very heavy work*, objects more than 100 lb must be lifted and objects more than 50 lb are carried.

561. The answer is E (all). *(Feutz Harter, Pain Digest 1:13–16, 1991.)* Only objective information within the personal knowledge of the physician should be documented. Avoid writing opinions or characterizations of events unless there is objective evidence to support the subjective statement. The time of entry in a medical record should be noted. Other important times may be included in the body of the entry. Legible writing is essential. Inability to read one's own handwriting can create negligence. Only approved abbreviations should be used. This is required by the Joint Commission on Accreditation of Health Care Organizations as well as by many states. If another health care provider could not interpret an abbreviation and harm came to the patient, the physician who used the unauthorized abbreviation could be sued for malpractice.

562. The answer is E (all). *(Feutz Harter, Pain Digest 1:13–16, 1991.)* The five elements necessary for informed consent are as follows:

1. Statement of the nature and purpose of the proposed treatment.
2. Statement of the expected outcome and the likelihood of success.
3. Statement of the material risks.
4. Statement of alternative procedures or treatments and supporting information regarding those alternatives.
5. Statement of the effect of no treatment, the effect on the prognosis, and material risks associated with no treatment.

563. The answer is E (all). *(AMA Guides to the Evaluation of Permanent Impairment, pp 1–2.)* All the statements listed apply to the term *handicap* as defined in the AMA guidelines. It is the physician's responsibility to evaluate a patient's health status and determine the degree of impairment. If the physician also has the ability to assess the patient's activities and need for assistive devices to perform those activities, an opinion regarding the degree of disability or handicap may be given as well.

564. The answer is B (1,3). *(AMA Guides to the Evaluation of Permanent Impairment, pp 1–2.)* Impairment is a medical condition specifically related to a disease process. It is expressed as a percentage of the body as a whole and may be defined as the derangement or loss of use of any body part, system, or function. Disability relates to employment or activities of daily living and is characterized as temporary, permanent, partial, or total.

Bibliography

American Medical Association (AMA): *Guides to the Evaluation of Permanent Impairment*, 4/e. Chicago, American Medical Association, 1994.

American Society of Regional Anesthesia (ASRA): *Comprehensive Review of Pain Management*. Naperville, IL, American Society of Regional Anesthesia, 1994.

Anastasio D: Current practices for release of medical information. *J Am Med Rec Assoc* 61:52–61, 1990.

Barolat G, Zeme S, Ketak B: Multifactorial analysis of epidural spinal cord stimulation. *Stereotact Funct Neurosurg* 56:77–103, 1991.

Bonica JJ (ed): *The Management of Pain*, 2/e, vols 1 and 2. Philadelphia, Lea & Febiger, 1990.

Braga PC: Calcitonin and its antinociceptive activity: Animal and human investigations 1975–1992. *Agents Actions* 41:121–131, 1994.

Broseta J, Barbera J, de Vera JA, et al: Spinal cord stimulation in peripheral arterial disease: A cooperative study. *J Neurosurg* 64:71–80, 1986.

Brown DL: *Atlas of regional anesthesia*. Philadelphia, Saunders, 1992.

Campbell JN, Meyer RA, Raja SN: Is nociceptor activation by alpha-1 adrenoreceptors the culprit in sympathetically-maintained pain? *APS Journal* 1:3–11, 1992.

Capan LM, Miller SM, Turndorf H (eds): *Trauma: Anesthesia and Intensive Care*. Philadelphia, Lippincott, 1991.

Cheshire WP, Abashian SW, Mann JD: Botulinum toxin in the treatment of myofascial pain syndrome. *Pain* 59:65–69, 1994.

Cousins MJ, Bridenbaugh PO (eds): *Neural blockade in Clinical Anesthesia and the Management of Pain*, 2/e. Philadelphia, Lippincott, 1987.

Ferrante FM, VadeBoncouer TR (eds): *Postoperative Pain Management* New York, Churchill Livingston, 1993.

Feutz Harter S: Special malpractice problems for the pain management specialist. *Pain Digest* 1:13–16, 1991.

Fishbain DA, Rosomoff HL, Rosomoff RS: Drug abuse, dependence, and addiction in chronic pain patients. *Clin J Pain* 8:77–75, 1992.

Gilman AG, Rall TW, Nies AS, Taylor P (eds): *Goodman and Gilman's The Pharmacological Basis of Therapeutics*, 8/e. New York, McGraw-Hill, 1990.

Greene P, Fahn S, Brin H, et al: Double-blind, placebo controlled trial of botulinum toxin injections for the treatment of spasmodic torticollis. *Neurology* 40:1213–1218, 1990.

Griffith RA, Schneider DC: Safeguarding the confidentiality of medical and mental health records. *Med Staff Couns* 5:31–37, 1991.

Guidelines for prescribers of controlled substances: A joint statement of the Drug Enforcement Administration (DEA) and the DEA/Practitioners Working Committee. *Federation Bulletin: Journal of Medical Licensure and Discipline* 67:47–50, 1980.

Jacox A, Carr DB, Payne R, et al: Management of cancer pain. Clinical practice guideline No. 9. *Agency for Health Care Policy and Research* (AHCPR) Publication No. 94-0592. Rockville, MD. US Department of Health and Human Services, Public Health Service, March 1994.

Jaffe JH: "Drug addiction and drug abuse." In Gilman AG, Rall TW, Nies AS, Taylor P (eds): *The Pharmacological Basis of Therapeutics*, 8/e. New York, McGraw-Hill, 1990, pp 522–573.

Joranson DE, Cleeland CS, Weissman DE, et al: Opioids for chronic cancer and non-cancer pain: A survey of state medical board members. *Federation Bulletin: Journal of Medical Licensure and Discipline* 79:15–49, 1992.

Livengood JM, Young CM, Parris WCW: Implications of multiple personality disorder for treatment of chronic pain. *Pain Digest* 4:191–194, 1994.

North RB, Kidd DH, Zahurak M, et al: Spinal cord stimulation for chronic intractable pain: Experience over two decades. *Neurosurgery* 32:384–394, discussion 394–395, 1993.

Physicians' Desk Reference (PDR), 49/e. Montvale, NJ, Medical Economics, 1995.

Raj PP (ed); *Practical Management of Pain*, 2/e. St. Louis, Mosby–Year Book, 1992.

Ramamurthy S, Rogers JN (eds): *Decision Making in Pain Management*. St. Louis, Mosby–Year Book, 1993.

Ready BL, Edwards WT (eds): *Management of Acute Pain: A Practical Guide*. Seattle, International Association for the Study of Pain Publications, 1992.

Robinson RG, Preston DF, Schiefelbein M, et al: Strontium-89 therapy for the palliation of pain due to osseous metastases. *JAMA* 274:420–424, 1995.

Savage SR: Addiction in the treatment of pain: Significance, recognition, and management. *J Pain Symptom Management* 8:265–278, 1993.

Shoemaker WC, Thompson WL, Holbrook PR (eds): *Textbook of Critical Care Medicine*. Philadelphia, Saunders, 1984.

Stoelting RK: *Pharmacology and Physiology in Anesthetic Practice*. Philadelphia, Lippincott, 1987.

Tollison CD (ed): *Handbook of Chronic Pain Management*. Baltimore, Williams & Wilkins, 1989.

Wall PD, Melzack R (eds): *Textbook of Pain*, 3/e. New York, Churchill Livingstone, 1994.

Wiener SL: *Differential Diagnosis of Acute Pain by Body Region*. New York, McGraw-Hill, 1993.

ISBN 0-07-052079-8

KAHN/PAIN MANAGEMENT